A HEALTHIER You!

D0168103

Insight Publishing
Sevierville, Tennessee

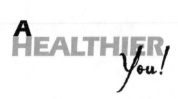

Published by Insight Publishing Company
P.O. Box 4189
Sevierville, Tennessee 37864

10 9 8 7 6 5 4 3 2

Printed in The United States

ISBN: 1-932863-63-X

Table Of Contents

A Message From The Publisher

This book is more than a collection of interviews from men and women who care about your health and well being. *A Healthier You* is an intimate introduction into the lives and hearts of eighteen very special people, people who are passionate about living and living well! Through their stories, and the lessons they've learned, you can discover new insights into your own physical and emotional health.

I've learned that advice from a trusted friend with whom you have a shared experience is usually advice worth considering. The woman fighting chronic pain can trust a friend who is battling the same demons and who recently discovered a therapy that helps. A daughter with cancer can find comfort from her mom, a cancer survivor. The overweight man struggling to improve his health through diet and exercise is open to the counsel from a close friend who has lost 50 pounds and kept off the weight.

I hope you'll consider these eighteen professionals trustworthy advisors. Their insights and strategies deserve careful consideration. If something they recommend sounds reasonable and might help you improve your health, I hope you will talk to those whom you trust and consider implementing their ideas.

All of us at Insight Publishing have grown to appreciate this wonderful group of contributors who have offered us tips to becoming *A Healthier You!*

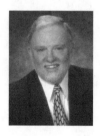

Interviews conducted by:

David E. Wright
President, International Speakers Network

Chapter 1

Sen No Sen — Your Sixth Sense
& The Key to Living a Safer, Happier Life

Mel H. Abraham,
CPA, CVA, ABV, ASA

In this chapter, we will explore a variety of different elements associated with our personal safety, our loved ones' safety, and the safety of society. It is unfortunate that we live in a time when we must consciously think and plan for the possibility of violence to occur within our lifetime. Unfortunate as it may be, it is however a reality we must live with and deal with. Hopefully over time we will begin to take the appropriate steps to lessen the impact of violence on all of our lives.

I know I've taken some strong positions in this chapter as well as making some strong statements, however, when it comes to our loved ones, ourselves, and especially our children, we cannot take it lightly. We must deal with it strictly, resolutely, and absolutely, without any doubt, without any hesitation, and with all the determination necessary to continue to thrive and survive these times.

We live in a society that at times unfortunately preys on or victimizes the young, women, children, the naïve or even those who just happen to be in the wrong place at the wrong time. In many cases, the perpetrator or attacker is someone who's known to the victims. It is our responsibility and duty as a society to protect our loved ones and ourselves as well as to protect those who are unable to protect themselves or who are unaware of societal dangers.

As we strive to live a healthier life, we find we must also search out a safer life in a society that experiences a number of episodes of violence unprecedented compared with previous historical times. Unfortunately most people live their lives in a state of denial or with the belief that "this stuff" won't happen in their neighborhood. Well, let's take a step back and look at some statistics from the various studies that have been done.

- 25 percent of college women surveyed said they were victims of rape or attempted rape.
- 85 percent of rapes on campuses are acquaintance- or date-rape.
- 73 percent of those forced to have sex failed to recognize their experience as rape.
- 90 percent of all campus rapes occur when either the assailant or the victim has used alcohol.
- 70 percent of college students admit to having engaged in sexual activity primarily as a result of being under the influence of alcohol, or to having sex. only because they were not sober enough to refuse.
- 84 percent of assaulted women knew their assailant.
- 40 percent of men stated they would rape under certain circumstances.
- 84 percent of college men who committed rape said that what they did was definitely not rape.
- A woman is actually assaulted every two minutes in the United States.
- There's an attempted abduction every six minutes in the United States.
- One in twelve high-schoolers is threatened or injured with a weapon each year.
- People between the ages of twelve and twenty-four the highest risk of being the victim of violence.
- Between the ages of fifteen to twenty-four years old, murder is the second leading cause of death. For African-American youths, murder is the number one cause of death.
- Every five minutes, a child is arrested in America for committing a violent crime.

- Gun related violence takes the life of an American child every three hours.
- Since 1960 teen suicide has tripled.
- At least 160,000 children fail to attend school every day because they fear an attack or intimidation by other students.

These are eye-opening and staggering statistics in any society, let alone a civilized society; and these statistics do not include the impact of child abuse, pedophile attacks or domestic violence. Do you realize that the average child molester has victimized between fifty and 150 children before ever being arrested?

Unfortunately, the conventional mindset is that violence is someone else's problem. People have taken the attitude that violence surrounds us and is part of our everyday life. We need to make it clear that just because violence happens to be prevalent in society today it is neither right nor appropriate, and we as a society must take a stand to reverse the trend of increasing violence. Clearly, you can see from the statistics above that violence is society's problem and until society becomes intolerant and resolute in their determination to eliminate violence, it will continue to grow like a cancer or plague, terrorizing everyone it comes in contact with.

It is important to consider that violence does not limit its impact to the perpetrator and victim. Be certain that the loss of life, be it psychological or physical, has a ripple effect throughout generations well beyond the victim. You have children who are losing fathers and mothers and siblings who are losing brothers and sisters. As this happens, not only does violence impact the current generation but it also impacts future generations. In many cases, through the loss of a child, it eliminates all potential descendents beyond that child. No longer can we live in a mindset or belief that the police will handle it, or the criminal justice system will handle it, or that other experts will handle it.

Our law enforcement agencies are overburdened, outnumbered, and in some cases outgunned. Likewise, our justice system does an abysmal job, at best, of justly trying and incarcerating these predators. Too many times a predator is allowed to roam the streets to continue to prey on innocent people because of some technicality or issue that was not resolved properly at trial.

I know of a case where a man who had a history of violence and confrontations with the law as well as infractions involving the numerous firearms he possessed was allowed to go free after brutally and without reason shooting a seventeen-year-old boy in the head with a forty-four Magnum while under the influence of alcohol. The courts refused to allow any discussion as to his past acts in considering this man's propensity for violence and his pattern of negligence, alcohol abuse, and disdain for society that had been a habitual problem. Instead they allowed him to walk free, with impunity, without justice, and without punishment after killing an innocent youth who was his mother's only child. Further, when and if a predator is incarcerated, our penal system does a disastrous job of rehabilitation with these criminals. Time and time again, we see criminals committing violent crimes shortly after being released from jail.

One such criminal was Joe Gray. With thirteen prior arrests and outstanding probation issues Gray was allowed back on the streets, where he was able to kidnap and murder an eleven-year-old girl.

We as members of society, as parents, as children, and as members of the human race have a responsibility as well as a right to live a life free from the anxiety, free from the psychological scars, and the erosion of our future caused by violence or even the apprehension of violence.

So What Is The Solution?

Our solution is not going to come from some outside force or some government agency. It is going to be developed internally through developing our sixth sense. I am not talking about some sort of extra sensory perception. I am talking about, simply "awareness." The definition of "aware" is "...having knowledge or cognizance..." or, "vigilant or watchful." The reality is we need to raise our awareness level.

In order to raise our awareness and develop this sixth sense, we need to raise our consciousness as to how violence is committed, how victims are selected, and the ploys and toys used by these predators.

The Japanese martial arts system is a self-defense method that distinguishes between various strategies that involve different elements of *timing*. Generally speaking, you can wait for the attacker to fully launch his assault, which is blocked and followed by your own counterattack. This is known as *"Go No Sen"*—"after method." Alternatively, just as the attacker commits himself to an attack, you seize the initiative to counter before he has the chance of completing his intention. This is the "before method," or "*Sen No Sen*"—the act of intercepting an advancing attack with a decisive counter before the active attack begins.

Why Sen No Sen?

Applied to our societal safety, Sen No Sen represents identifying and understanding threats as well as the key ploys to more readily anticipate a potential harmful situation before it ever becomes an actual physical problem.

In my three decades as a martial arts professional, personal protection, and defensive tactics consultant, I have learned many ways to physically protect myself as well as my loved ones. In fact and unfortunately, I have had the need on a few occasions to use my skills, including successfully defending myself during two separate knife attacks. At the time I felt I was well trained and my students were well trained. However, it wasn't until one of my students, a beautiful sixteen-year-old girl—a black belt and a superb fighter—came to me to tell me the story of how she was assaulted. You see, I never worried about her in a physical altercation because she could handle herself very well. In fact, she could beat most guys I know! However, what I did not anticipate was what happens if we are not able to physically defend ourselves because we never had the opportunity to?

This young lady was attending a party with some friends (a seemingly safe environment). Someone put something in her drink and ultimately she woke up the next morning having been sexually assaulted, not recalling a thing, and blaming herself.

This unfortunate set of events made me realize that I failed her as an instructor. I also realized that though I have always taught our students and in my seminars around the country that fighting is a *last* resort, I needed to teach personal protection as a *first* resort. I failed her by not giving her the proper tools and skills—the Sen No Sen—to recognize what was happening and recognize potential threats before they became reality. This is the sixth sense—the art of heightened awareness and consciousness—we need to develop in ourselves and in our children.

It is my belief that few crimes are random and that most crimes are selective. In other words, these predators stalk their potential victims, hunt them down based on certain criteria, and if you fit their profile, you may become the victim.

So Where Do We Go from Here?

It is important to understand the "three legs of violence" and to further understand the detailed means in which a predator gets close to prey. Through this understanding, we can readily recognize a threatening situation before it completely unfolds and be better prepared to avoid or deal with the situation. Just like the three legs of a stool, if one leg is missing, the stool cannot stand. In the same way, if all three legs of violence in any potential crime scenario are not present there is a much lower likelihood of success for the predator.

By controlling at least one leg of violence, it is difficult if not impossible for us to be victimized.

The three legs of violence are:

- Opportunity
- Privacy
- Control

Think of this in the context of an abduction that happened in Century City, California. It involved a young lady who was an aspiring actress and model. One day at a mall she met a well-dressed and handsome man. He explained to her that he was a photographer and handed her a business card. They then set up a meeting so he could do a photo shoot of her. She went to a public location to meet him for the photo shoot. When she got there, he then took her with him to the actual location of the "supposed" photo shoot. She was never seen alive again.

This is a very typical scenario. It seems to be repeated over and over again across the country. So how do the three legs of violence apply to this situation? First, once the man realized she was an aspiring actress or model, this gave him the first leg— *opportunity*. Through exploiting her desire to become a model, he was able to convince her to have a second meeting. The second leg of violence happened at the initial meeting site. The first meeting site seemed public enough and safe enough—a public location where people would be around. However, the second meeting gave him *privacy* with her and put him in the position to gain the last and third leg of violence—*control*. Once he successfully moved the meeting from the initial public place, he achieved all three legs of violence and had control of the situation. He effectively cut her off from any lifeline to anyone who knew where she was or where she was going and from any trace or way to trace where she was finally taken.

At any time during this process, had she understood the three legs of violence and held back at least one leg she would still be with us today. Now, you may ask how I can be so sure? The answer comes from another young lady, who was approached by the same man two weeks earlier. In her case, she set up the meeting. She in fact, went to the meeting. However when he tried to relocate the meeting, she refused to go. He in fact, tried to physically take her and she fought back. The smart actions of this girl kept her alive and she was able to help the police identify this man who murdered the other young lady.

We must be vigilant with the opportunities we provide strangers in allowing them to gain privacy and control of us and we must be vigilant to realize the danger we put ourselves in. Had she for a moment stepped back to look at the context in which this scenario was unfolding, she would've had a better understanding of the potential danger she was facing. The context in this case was that this was a stranger—someone she did not know—he walked up to her in a mall one day and handed her a business card saying he wanted to photograph her. Without understanding clearly what the context is in which these seemingly chance meetings come about, we do not see reality and cannot have the heightened awareness or vision—the Sen No Sen—to avoid a dangerous situation.

The other element that we need to be mindful of are the *4 Rules of Safety*. These rules of safety, provide us and our children a lifestyle that promotes safety, awareness and confidence. The four rules are as follows:

1. **Create Safe Habits** - This element is no different than putting the seat belt on when you get in the car or locking the door when you get home. It is not that you're acting out of panic or paranoia. It is plainly a safe habit to get into and just like any other habits, the more we do it, the more natural it becomes.

2. **Be Aware not Afraid** - We need to walk through life with our head up, our eyes opened and constantly examining our environment and surroundings. Remember, these violent acts are not random rather they are selective and as such by being aware with a confident air about you, reduces substantially the possibility of you becoming a victim. Whereas if you walk through life in a state of paranoia or fear this will be

> sensed by a predator and raise the possibility of you becoming a victim.

3. **Intuition** – This is that little voice inside of your head or that gut feeling that you get when things just don't seem right. Two things to consider with intuition are that it is always in response to some stimulus in your environment. In other words, something outside of you is causing you to feel this way, to feel apprehension or fear. The second element about intuition is that it always has your best interests in mind. So, if it is reacting to some outside stimulus and it has your best interest in mind then we need to learn to listen to that voice or that gut feeling. Even if we are wrong, we are safe.

4. **If In Doubt, Get Out** – This one is pure and simple, if you have a doubt about a situation or feel uncomfortable, simply get out, leave. Do not concern yourself with what others will think, or what others say, simply get out, if you have a doubt.

With a raised level of awareness and consciousness, you are in a better position to identify and recognize the variety of strategies or tactics typically used by predators to get close to their prey. Gavin de Becker has best enumerated these strategies and tactics. The key to understanding these is to view them in their proper context, and to be consciously aware that the strategy or tactic is being put into play against you. By doing so, we just might see the "wolf in sheep's clothing."

Forced teaming—Perpetrators using this tactic will seek to create an attachment or partnership—a sense of "we"—with the intended victim. This allows them to get close and create a sense of trust. An example of this would be in a situation where, for instance, you are purchasing dog food at the grocery store and a stranger approaches you and says, "Oh, we have a dog, do we?" The use of the term "we" in this context subconsciously creates a familiarity between two people that in reality does not exist.

Charm and niceness—Our culture has a false belief that someone who is polite and charming is a "good" person. Perpetrators use this strategy to get victims to lower their guard. In the story I told you earlier a man posing as a photographer who was charming and handsome used that strategy. What is important to consider is to view charm as a verb and not an adjective. What I mean is, if you find yourself thinking, "My! He's charming!" You ought to follow it up with the question, "What is he trying to charm me out of?" You see, by considering "charm" a verb, it places a different context on the interaction between you and the other person.

Too many details—When attempting to mislead a victim, perpetrators will often use talk and provide "too many details" to appear open and friendly. A skillful liar uses detail to create the appearance of openness, honesty, and truth or familiarity with the victim. Typically, this tactic entails talking about unrelated information in order to bring more depth to a conversation, which in turn may raise your comfort level since it gets you to believe you know more about this person than you really do.

Typecasting—This is a highly manipulative tactic. The perpetrator uses a slight insult to get the victim to feel the need to disprove the accusation by cooperating. Unfortunately, we as individuals—especially women—have a desire to be viewed in a certain light and in many cases a predator may make a slight insult to show contempt about how your values, standards, or principles are viewed. The immediate reaction will be to disprove the comment by in fact, allowing the predator to manipulate you into doing exactly what they want you to do.

Loan sharking—The predator using this tactic will often do an unsolicited favor for the victim in order to make the victim feel obligated or indebted in some way. This can be as simple as helping carry a package to the car. Unfortunately, the concept of reciprocity comes into play here. Reciprocity is a long-time negotiating tactic in which one party does a seemingly small favor for another, which causes the other to feel obligated to repay the favor. To allow more access and time with the intended victim, a predator may use this tactic. Through this tactic a predator may find it easier to move through the three legs of violence.

Unsolicited promise—In this tactic, the predator will often make an unsolicited promise to reassure the victim or quiet natural suspicions. *An unsolicited promise in any setting is a way to convince you to do something he wants!* This typically plays out in a situation where the predator believes you might have some distrust or suspicion about them. As a result they may make a statement such as, "I'll just make the one phone call and then be out of here. I promise."

Discounting the word "No"—The word "No" IS A COMPLETE SENTENCE! There is no explaining necessary—ever. Anything further softens the meaning. Unfortunately, to many this is simply the beginning of a negotiation. YOU DO NOT NEGOTIATE THE WORD "NO!" Too often we don't want to appear cold or callous, so we temper our true meaning by softening it with an explanation. However, if you mean no, then that is all you need to say with no need to explain any further. This comes into play in many cases—especially with young adults at parties—during parties when others are trying to convince you to take a drink. How this works is that at the beginning, you will typically say no to a whole drink. This leads to negotiation until they wear you down to the point of saying yes or getting you to say yes to a lesser level of commitment such as a taste instead of a full drink. Once they have moved you to this point, they have broken down your barriers and they will continue to infringe more and more on your comfort zone. It's important that you *not* be concerned about any stranger you just met or what they think of you and your reaction to him or her. To the extent you are uncomfortable, or unsure or uneasy, you need to simply say no and walk away. If they are disrespectful enough, and inconsiderate enough to continue, you need to escalate your resolve and succinctly, confidently, and clearly state your position. Discuss the matter no further.

As you continue to familiarize yourself with the strategies and tactics used by predators to gain access to our comfort zone, to bring a level of familiarity to a situation that doesn't belong, and to raise the level of comfort that should not exist, you will be better prepared to view things in the proper context. When you do, you will be able to see potential hazards before they materialize— the art of *Sen No Sen*—the art of heightened awareness and consciousness.

Now that we've set the stage and discussed some fundamentals of threat recognition, I want to take a moment to deal with some very specific issues that impact our lives and families, including stalking, bullying, and abuse.

Stalking

Stalking is a "willful course of conduct" involving repeated or continuing harassment of another individual that would cause a reasonable person to feel terrorized, frightened, intimidated, threatened, "harassed," or molested. It actually causes the victim to feel threatened

Stalking can take many forms. According to the anti-stalking laws, a person can be charged with stalking for willfully and repeatedly contacting another individual without permission. Under these laws, assailants could be charged with stalking for repeatedly:

- Following or appearing within the sight of another.
- Approaching or confronting another individual in a public or private place.
- Appearing at the work place or residence of another.
- Entering or remaining on an individual's property.
- Contacting by telephone.
- Sending mail or electronic mail.

Remember, you neither wanted nor deserved to be stalked. *You* are the victim, not the criminal. Suggestions of what to do if stalked are listed below. Every situation is different, so there are no set guidelines. Use your own judgment as to what actions to take.

Make sure you have communicated a definite "NO" to the stalker, not just brushed them off. Then end *all* communication with them (i.e., do not initiate any kind of contact).

If you are being stalked, immediately contact your local police department and let them know that you are a victim of stalking, *whether or not* you plan to file formal charges. If possible, you can ask the department to increase patrols in your area; or better yet, get to know the officers on your beat. Be especially careful if the police suggest a restraining order, as this is a response to the stalker and you have no way of knowing who will and who won't obey the order, or if the order will be a trigger event that will push the stalker into escalating their attempts or to violence in reaction.

Make sure your employer, friends, and family members are aware of the situation. The more eyes watching your back, the safer you will be.

Build your case against the stalker by providing the police with as much of the following as you can:

- Documentation (personal journal or diary) of the stalker's activities.
- Taped recording(s) of threatening telephone calls.
- Videotape of stalker's actions.
- Basic identifying information (i.e., license plate number, make of car, personal appearance).
- List of contacts with the stalker (i.e., date, time, place, what was said, letters/calls received).

Abuse or Domestic Violence

Many people in society believe that battering and abuse is extremely rare. Unfortunately battering is extremely common. The F.B.I. estimates that a woman is battered every fifteen seconds. National studies indicate that at least one in ten American women each year are abused by the men in their lives. In fact, half of all marriages involve at least one episode of violence between spouses. At least 1.8 million of these women are severely beaten every year. The National Centers for Disease Control and Prevention (CDC) has reported that attacks by husbands on wives result in more injuries requiring medical treatment than rapes, muggings, and auto accidents combined. Other studies show that forty percent of all murdered women are killed by their husbands or lovers. These statistics are shocking. However, the actual extent of the problem may be even worse since only an estimated one in ten episodes is even reported to the police. Domestic violence is this country's most under reported crime.

Additionally, many people believe that domestic abuse is a "lower class" phenomenon. Again, this is untrue. Even though many people would like to believe this, the truth is that men who abuse their partners are from every race, religion, and socio-economic background. Women have reported attacks by their partners who are doctors, clergymen, lawyers, police officers, judges, therapists, administrators, teachers, etc.

Abuse will typically follow a cycle that begins with a *"tension-building phase,"* which leads to the *"abuse phase,"* which is followed by the *"honeymoon phase"* until the process starts all over again. This cycle can last a matter of days to a matter of years. During each of these phases both the victim and the abuser will demonstrate certain traits as follows:

Abuser	Victim
Tension Phase	
Jealousy	Calming Techniques
Isolation of Victim	Minimizing
Rule Changing	Anger Suppression
Name Calling	Fatigue
Dominating	Confusion
Threats	Self-doubt
	Withdrawal
	Fear
Abuse Phase	
Anger	Fear
Uncontrolled Tension	Anger
Assault on Victim	May Call Police
Exhaustion	May Flee
Honeymoon Phase	
Apologies	Guilt
Promises	Hope
Insecurities	Loneliness
Loving	May Return
Dependency	Low Self-esteem
	Dependency
	Deceived

It is important for the victim to understand this process, to be realistic and honest with himself or herself at the beginning stages of a relationship to recognize the various characteristics and indicators that the individual is a potential abuser. By understanding the characteristics and realistically and honestly considering them, victims can increase their ability to avoid a potentially volatile and deadly situation before it ever occurs. In fact, to be able to recognize these traits at early stages of a relationship will allow you to remove yourself before you get too involved or it becomes a problem. Again Sen No Sen. Some characteristics to look for include the following:

- *Jealousy:* At the beginning of a relationship, an abuser will always say that jealousy is a sign of love. Jealousy has nothing to do with love. It is a sign of possessiveness and lack of trust. The abuser will question the partner about who s/he talks to, accuse the partner of flirting, or be jealous of time s/he spends with family, friends, or children. As the jealousy progresses, the abuser may call frequently during the day or drop by unexpectedly. The abusive partner may refuse to let his/her partner work for fear s/he will meet someone else. The abuser may check car mileage or ask friends to watch their partner for them in their absence.

- *Controlling Behavior:* At first, the abuser will say this behavior is because s/he is concerned for the victim's safety, her/his need to use her/his time well, or her/his need to make good decisions. The abuser will be angry if the partner is "late" coming back from the store or an appointment. The abuser will question the partner closely about where s/he went, whom s/he talked to. As this behavior worsens, the abuser may not let the partner make personal decisions about the house, what to wear, or going to church or other outside activities. The abuser may keep all the money or even make the partner ask permission to leave the house or room.

- *Quick Involvement:* Many victims of domestic violence dated or knew their abuser for less than six months before they were married, engaged, or living together. The abusive partner comes on like a whirlwind, claiming, "You are the only person I could ever talk to," or, "I have never felt loved like this by anyone." S/he will pressure the potential partner to commit to the relationship in such a way that later the partner may feel very guilty or that s/he is "letting the partner down" if s/he wants to slow down involvement or break it off.

- *Unrealistic Expectations:* Abusive people will expect their partner to meet all their needs; s/he expects the partner to be the perfect spouse, parent, lover, and friend. The abusive partner will say things like, "If you love me..." or, "I am all you need," or, "You are all I need." That victim is supposed to take care of everything for him/her emotionally and in the home.

- *Isolation:* The abusive person tries to cut the victim off from all resources. If the victim has friends of the opposite sex, s/he is "fooling around." If s/he has same sex friends, s/he is "homosexual." If s/he is close to family, s/he is "tied to the apron strings." The abuser accuses people who are in support of the victim of "causing trouble." The abuser may want to live out in the country without a phone; s/he may not let their partner use a car (or have one that is reliable), or s/he may try to keep the victim from working or going to school.

- *Blames Others For Problems:* If the abuser is chronically unemployed, someone is always doing him/her wrong, or is out to get him/her. The abuser may make mistakes and then blame the partner for upsetting him/her and keeping him/her from concentrating on work. The abuser will tell the partner s/he is at fault for almost anything that goes wrong.

- *Blames Others for Feelings:* An abuser will make statements to the partner such as, "You make me mad," or, "you are hurting me by not doing what I want you to do," or, "I cannot help being angry." S/he really makes the decision about what s/he thinks or feels, but will use feelings to manipulate the partner. Harder to catch are claims that, "you make me happy," and "you control how I feel."

- *Hypersensitivity:* An abuser is easily insulted, and will claim his/her feelings are "hurt" when really s/he is very mad or s/he takes the slightest setbacks as personal attacks. The abusive partner will "rant and rave" about the injustice of things that have happened that are really just part of living such as being asked to work overtime, getting a traffic ticket, being told some behavior is annoying, or being asked to help with chores.

- *Cruelty to Animals or Children:* Abusers may punish animals brutally or be insensitive to their pain or suffering. S/he may expect children to be capable for doing things beyond their ability (spanks a two-year-old for wetting a diaper) or s/he may tease children or young brothers and sisters until they cry. The abuser may not want children to eat at the table or expect to keep them in their room all evening while s/he is home.

- *"Playful" Use of Force in Sex:* This kind of person may like to throw the partner down and hold her/him down during sex. S/he may want to act out fantasies during sex where the partner is helpless. The abuser is letting the partner know that the idea of rape is exciting. He/she may show little concern about whether the partner wants to have sex and uses sulking or anger to manipulate her/him into compliance. The abuser may start having sex with the partner while s/he is sleeping, or demand sex when s/he is ill or tired.
- *Verbal Abuse:* In addition to saying things that are meant to be cruel and hurtful, this can be seen when the abuser degrades the partner, cursing her/him, running down any of her/his accomplishments. The abuser will tell the partner that s/he is stupid and unable to function without him/her. This may involve waking the partner up to verbally abuse her/him or not letting her/him go to sleep.
- *Rigid Sex Roles:* The abuser expects the partner to serve them; the abuser may say the partner must stay at home, that s/he must obey in all things, even things that are criminal in nature. In heterosexual relationships, the abuser will see women as inferior to men, responsible for menial tasks, stupid, and unable to be a whole person without a relationship.
- *Dr. Jekyll and Mr. Hyde:* Many victims are confused by their abuser's "sudden" changes in mood—they may think the abuser has some special mental problem because one minute s/he is nice and the next s/he is exploding. Explosiveness and moodiness are typical of people who abuse their partners, and these behaviors are related to other characteristics like hypersensitivity.
- *Past Battering:* This person may say s/he has hit others in the past, but the other person "made him/her do it." The partner may hear from relatives or ex-intimate partners that the person is abusive. An abuser will beat any partner they are with if the partner is with him/her long enough for the violence to begin.
- *Threats of Violence:* This could include any threat of physical force meant to control the partner such as, "I'll slap your mouth off," or, "I will kill you," or, "I will break your neck."

Most people do not threaten their mates, but an abuser will try to excuse threats by saying "everybody talks like that."

- *Breaking or Striking Objects*: This behavior maybe used as a punishment (breaking loved possessions), but is mostly used to terrorize the partner into submission. The abuser may beat on the table with his/her fist; throw objects around or near the partner. Again, this is very remarkable behavior—not only is this a sign of extreme emotional immaturity, but there is great danger when someone thinks they have the "right" to punish or frighten their partner.
- *Any Force During an Argument:* This may involve a batterer holding the partner down, physically restraining her/him from leaving the room, and pushing or shoving. They may hold the victim against the wall and say, "you are going to listen to me!"

Do not make the unfortunate mistake that most people make—to believe they are different than the people who came before them in the relationship. To believe you will be treated any differently than other victims of the abuser during past relationships is both a naïve and dangerous mindset. To believe that the abuse only happened once and it won't happen again is again a naïve and dangerous mindset. No matter how charming, handsome, beautiful, or rich a person is; if they possess these abusive traits or if you have been a victimized by either verbal or physical abuse even once, you have no alternative but to get out immediately. It cannot and will not lead to anything positive. Get out before you can't get out.

As you prepare to move away from an abusive relationship, some additional safety precautions or considerations includes some of the following:

- Hide extra money, car keys and coil wire (for car).
- Hide important documents (i.e., marriage license, birth certificates, social security cards, school records, etc.) in a safe place so you can get to them in a hurry.
- Keep a bag/suitcase packed for emergency exits. Leave this with a trusted friend or relative.
- Plan for a place to go in case of an emergency such as a shelter, trusted friend, or relative's house.
- Have the phone number of the police department available (dial 911 for all emergency calls) and get the name/badge

number of the responding officer(s) should the need arise to call.

- Teach and encourage the children to go to a neighbor's house to call 911 during an abusive incident.
- If possible, have a special room in the house with an extra strong lock.
- Understand the cycle of violence so that you can recognize when a violent episode may occur; then take the children and leave the house at once.
- If attacked, go to the hospital for prompt medical attention; have the abuse documented as domestic violence on hospital records.
- Keep a record of injuries, including photographs, so that legal evidence can be produced to press charges and/or secure a Personal Protection Order (PPO).
- Have a special signal to use with neighbors, friends, or relatives with which to alert a call for help such as listening for screams, your lights flickering on and off, etc. When seeing those signals the neighbor, friend, or relative can then notify the police.
- If the survivor returns home to the joint residence and the abuser has been evicted, all locks should be changed immediately.
- Conduct daily routines at different times of day if possible. Utilize different grocery stores or shopping malls. Take alternate routes to work and schools.

Bullying

Have you ever met a bully? A bully is a male or female who acts mean or hurtful to others. Bullies pick on someone else as a way to get power, or to get their way, or to feel important.

Bullies sometimes hit, kick, or push to hurt people, and they sometimes use words to call names, tease, or scare them. A bully might say mean things about someone, grab a kid's stuff, make fun of someone, or leave a kid out of the group on purpose. Some bullies threaten people or try to make them do things they don't want to do.

Bullying is a big problem that affects lots of kids. Being bullied can make kids feel scared, sad, worried, or embarrassed. The stress of dealing with bullies can even make kids sick!

Some bullies are just looking for attention. They might think bullying is a way to be popular or a way to get what they want. Most bullies are trying to make themselves feel more important—when they pick on someone else; it makes them feel big and powerful.

Some bullies come from families where everyone is angry and shouting all the time. They may think that being angry, calling names, and pushing people around is a normal way to act. Some bullies are copying what they've seen someone else do. Some have been bullied themselves.

Sometimes a bully knows that what he or she is doing or saying hurts other people. But other bullies may not really know how hurtful their actions can be. Most bullies don't understand or care about the feelings of others.

Bullies often pick on someone they think they can have power over. They might pick on kids who get upset easily or who have trouble defending themselves. Getting a big reaction out of someone can make bullies feel like they have the power they want. Sometimes bullies pick on someone who is smarter than they are or different from them in some way. Sometimes bullies just pick on a kid for no reason at all.

We try to teach our students and parents promote the use of the "ASE Principles" ™ when dealing with bullying problems. The principles are:

- *Avert*—We avert conflict by raising our awareness of it by using the principle of Sen No Sen. As we become aware of these potential conflicts and we recognize them, we can avoid the situation altogether or try to prevent it before it begins.
- *Solve*—When we have been unsuccessful in averting the conflict and it has begun, then the second stage would be to solve it through the use of various nonviolent verbal skills—verbal jujitsu if you will. We will discuss a number of these further below.
- *Engage*—Lastly, if we are unsuccessful in averting or solving the conflict, then we may need to call on our physical personal safety skills to bring the conflict to an end as humanely as possible.

Here are some things to try if a bully bothers you:

- *Befriend*—Typically bullies become bullies because they were bullied once themselves. Even bullies need admiration and respect. Try to figure out a way to befriend the bully. Confront your fear and ask the bully for help such as how to play baseball for instance, or offer to help the bully with something you know how to do such as English homework.

- *Humor/Cleverness*—Try to make the bully laugh. By making the bully laugh you will throw him off guard. You may even want to make fun as long as you don't make fun of the bully. By doing so, you are taking a threatening situation and making it a funny one. Or through the use of distraction (cleverness comes in here) you may be able to get away.

- *Walk/Ignore*—Don't engage him—just walk away. This is an often neglected way to solve the problem. When you begin to walk away and ignore him, continue to do so, no matter what is being said.

- *Agree*—Agree with the bully. By agreeing with the bully you effectively take the energy out of his assault and there is no fight, which is what we are trying to avoid.

- *Refuse*—Refuse to fight. No matter what happens just say no.

- *Stand up*—Stand up to the bully face-to-face. Be careful with this strategy, as you can escalate the situation if done incorrectly or in the wrong circumstances.

- *Authority*—Seek out authority. Call a teacher, police officer, parent, or someone you know who can keep the bully from hurting you. This is not "tattling;" it is a way to stop a fight.

- *Reason*—Try and talk the bully out of it. If you have "the gift of gab," and you don't argue or get angry with him, you may just convince the bully not to hurt you.

- *Buddying*—Kids who are being bullied can use the buddy system. Make a plan to walk with a friend or two on the way to school, or recess, or lunch, or wherever you think you might meet the bully. Offer to do the same for a friend who's having trouble with a bully.

Internet/World Wide Web Safety

How could we exist without the Internet and the World Wide Web? These computer tools are how most of us keep in touch with friends, find homework support, research a cool place to visit, or find out the latest news. But just as there are millions of places to visit and things to do, there are also lots of places to waste time, even get into trouble. And, just like the rest of the world, there are some people who can take advantage of you—financially or physically.

You've probably heard stories about people who get into trouble in chat rooms. Because users can easily remain anonymous, chat rooms often attract people who are interested in more than just chatting. These people will sometimes ask visitors for information about themselves, their families, or where they live— information that shouldn't be given away.

Usually, people who request personal information like home addresses, phone numbers, and email addresses use this information to fill mailboxes and answering machines with advertisements. In some cases, though, predators may use this information to begin illegal or indecent relationships or to harm a person's or a family's well-being. It's rare, but it does happen.

Of course, the Internet is home to millions of places you can and should visit. Like a library, the Web can take you to the ends of the earth with the information it contains.

The key is to protect yourself while you "surf." Remain as anonymous as possible. That means keeping all private information private. Here are some examples of private information that you should never give out on the Internet:

- Full name
- Home address
- Phone number
- Social security numbers
- Passwords
- Names of family members
- Credit card numbers

Most credible people and companies will never ask for this type of information online. So if someone does, it's a red flag that they may be up to no good.

Think carefully before you create an email address or screen name. Web experts recommend that you use a combination of letters and numbers in both and that you don't identify whether you're male or female.

In chat rooms, use a nickname different from your screen name. That way, if you ever find yourself in a conversation that makes you uncomfortable, you can exit without having to worry that someone knows your screen name and can track you down via email. Some people who hang out with their friends online set up private chat rooms where only they and the people they invite can enter to chat. Check to see if your service provider (such as AOL, MSN, or Earthlink) offers this option.

Experts recommend that people keep online friendships in the virtual world. Meeting online friends face-to-face carries more risks than other types of friendships because it's so easy for people to pretend to be someone they're not when you can't see them or talk in person.

If you ever get involved in a chat room conversation that makes you feel uncomfortable or in danger for any reason, exit and tell a parent or other adult right away so they can report the incident. You can also report it to the website of the National Center for Missing and Exploited Children at www.missingkids.com. The organization has a form available there for reporting this type of incident called CyberTipline. They will then see the information is forwarded to law enforcement officials for investigation.

Cyber-bullying

Strangers are not the only people who can make you feel uncomfortable online. "Cyber-bullying" is a term that refers to cruel or bullying messages sent to you online. These might be from former friends or other people you know. They can be irritating and, in some cases, even frightening. If you get these kinds of messages online, it's often better to ignore them rather than answer them. Cyber-bullies, just like other bullies, may be angry or disturbed people and may be looking for attention or a reaction.

Fortunately, most people never experience cyber-bullying. But if you're getting cyber-bullied and ignoring it doesn't make it go away, getting help from a parent, school counselor, or another trusted adult may be a good idea. That's especially true if the cyber-bullying contains threats.

Fundamental Personal Protection Strategies

Personal safety requires four things: awareness, body language, self-esteem, and boundaries. Setting boundaries is probably the most important concept for you to understand. Knowing your boundaries before ever finding yourself in a compromising situation allows you to make better safety choices.

Boundaries come in two forms: physical boundaries which represent the space between you and another person, and emotional boundaries before ever finding yourself in a compromised situation which are lines you draw in terms of how you let other people treat you. For example, suppose you have a friend who constantly shares your secrets with other people. Unless you let h/her know how you feel, h/she will never know that your boundary has been invaded. However, if you do make your feelings known and the behavior that bothers you continues—your feelings are not being respected and your friend is overstepping that boundary.

Knowing your own boundaries puts you in a better position to recognize when you're in a potentially dangerous situation. If you're confident and you have a healthy self-esteem, you will more readily sense when trouble is near.

Using your awareness (Sen No Sen) and "verbal Jujitsu" are two common personal protection techniques. Have you ever been in a situation that just didn't feel right? Perhaps you were walking home alone one night from the bus stop and you had a weird feeling inside. That was your Sen No Sen at work telling you to be careful.

It's also important to understand the power of your voice. If you ever feel threatened, you should shout or scream to draw attention to the situation. It's even a good idea to practice speaking loudly (or yelling) so if you are ever in danger, you won't freeze up. Commands like "No!" "Go away!" or "Back off!" are excellent attention-getters if you feel threatened.

The National Crime Prevention Council offers the following personal safety tips to reduce your risk in a dangerous situation:

- If you're going to be out at night, travel in a group.
- Don't take shortcuts, especially at night.
- Be aware of your surroundings, and pay particular attention to possible hiding places such as stairways, alleyways, and bushes.

- Be sure your body language shows a sense of confidence and purpose.
- When riding on public transportation, sit near the driver or conductor and stay awake. Remember, attackers are looking for vulnerable targets.
- If someone begins to follow you, try to make it to a safe area, such as a police station, gas station, or other public place. If necessary, scream or yell as you run away to draw attention to the pursuer.
- If all else fails, it may be necessary to use physical force to protect yourself. However, you should first determine if fighting is really your *only* option. If possible, you should try to get away from the dangerous situation to a safe location where someone can help you. But if a person ignores boundaries you've set, blocks your path to safety, or if your Sen No Sen tells you something is wrong, you may have to fight.

There are five elements in a personal protection situation. You need to know what they are, when to use them, when not to use them, how to perform them and even what to do if they fail or backfire. The five include:

- Compliance
- Escape and Evasion
- De-escalation
- Defiance/Assertiveness
- Fighting Back

The one you choose is based on your assessment of the situation. Each of them is built on beliefs about predatory situations. For example, your belief about what is and isn't important enough to fight and risk injury for will determine whether you should comply or resist the demands of an assailant. A belief that an assailant is in search of a passive, compliant victim may cause you to challenge the assailant's demands and send him looking for a more cooperative target. Our beliefs determine our behavior. You need to consider each of the above strategies and think about what you believe to be true about personal protection situations.

Ultimately, a personal protection system teaches you what to do and why and how to do it. Your ability to defend yourself lies in doing the right thing right the right way at the right time. However, once you've decided to defend yourself or your loved ones, you need to act quickly, decisively and without conscience. You need to attack vital areas and weak areas of the body. This includes the usual strikes to the eyes, groin area, knees, or neck. However, it also includes nerve centers around the body. There are effectively 361 pressure points we can use to defend ourselves. It takes the appropriate training and practice to engage in a self-defense situation and readily access these points. Whether you are attacking general vital areas such as the eyes or nerve centers, it is very important to practice in advance—it is only through repetition and practice will you be able to use this kind of self-defense in a high stress conflict situation. Without repetition your body will not have the proper programming (i.e., "muscle memory") to react appropriately when an attack occurs. This is partly because of the physiological reactions of the body to stress as well as the "adrenaline dump" that occurs when the body goes into survival mode.

During a personal protection encounter the body can go into a phobic-scale response with disastrous results if we have not been properly trained through "stress inoculation" training or "adrenal stress" training to control the body's natural physiological response to an attack. This is done through continuous "stimulus response" training to the point that the body moves without thought—no different than the thought processes you use daily to get food on your fork and bring the food to your mouth. Through repetitive "stimulus response" you have been able to train the body to move without conscious thought. It is through this same type of repetitive "stimulus response" training while in a high or peak emotional state that anchors the immediate response into the threads of your being so you can instantly respond without thought and without panic or freezing.

Once you begin your defense, you should not and *cannot* stop until you are clearly safe. Then and only then should you cautiously move away from your assailant. Be careful at this moment, as it has been said that the most vulnerable time in combat is immediately following a successful engagement. This is primarily due to the fact that many soldiers will let down their guard, believing the engagement has ended and they are not prepared for a second wave of attack.

In conclusion, I want reiterate my opening. In this chapter, we have explored a variety of different elements associated with our personal safety, our loved ones' safety, and the safety of society. It is unfortunate that we live in a time when we must consciously think and plan for the possibility of violence to occur within our lifetime. Unfortunate as it may be, the threat of physical harm is however a reality we must live with, deal with, and hopefully over time begin to take appropriate steps to lessen its impact on our lives.

I realize I've taken some strong positions in this chapter as well as making some strong statements, however, when it comes to our loved ones, ourselves, and especially our children, we cannot take violence lightly. We must deal with it strictly, resolutely, and absolutely, without any doubt, without any hesitation, and with all the determination necessary to continue to thrive and survive during these times.

Remember in the words of Anthony Robbins, "Life is a gift, and it offers us the privilege, opportunity, and responsibility to give something back by becoming more."

I bid you a safe and glorious journey in your life with the ability to make a continued positive impact on the lives of all those you may touch!

About The Author

Mel H. Abraham, CPA, CVA, ABV, ASA

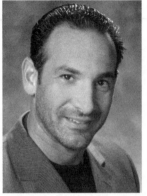

"Never before have we lived in a time where so many adversarial forces threaten our everyday existence. From identity theft and Internet scams, to corporate corruption, and property crimes, both our financial and personal security are constantly at risk."

Mel is a highly sought after expert (CPA) and a very successful entrepreneur with multiple businesses. Regularly called upon as a forensic expert in financial and valuation issues, he is also a nationally recognized and award-winning speaker having addressed professional conferences on local, state, and national levels. Mel's two-fold forté is providing strategies in financial risk management and in personal/physical, threat management, and self-protection. His clients span the country. In the personal protection realm, he is the creator of the highly requested presentation, "Bulletproof Boundaries"™—Safety & Success Strategies for an Unsafe World." This enlightening program provides intellectual tools for living with confidence and security in a risky world through awareness and recognition of threatening situations. Drawing on Mel's diverse expertise, this dynamic program addresses both personal safety and measures you can take to protect your financial corporate security against financial crimes. He has received numerous speaking awards and has authored numerous articles. His authoritative book, *Valuation Issues and Case Law Update—A Reference Guide*, has been released in a fourth edition. Recently, he was co-author of the business valuation industry's best selling book, *Financial Valuation: Applications and Models*, released last year by John Wiley & Sons, Inc. Three additional books will be released by mid-2005: *A Healthier You*, (with Deepak Chopra and Billy Blanks), *Masters of Success*, (with Ken Blanchard, Jack Canfield and John Christensen) and *Valuing Family Limited Partnerships*.

Mel H. Abraham
543 Country Club Drive, Suite B-543
Simi Valley, CA 93065
805.578.1515 • 805.293.8950 fax
mel@melabraham.com
www.melabraham.com

Special Feature

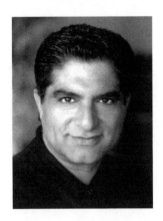

David Wright Interviews
Deepak Chopra
Internationally known leader in the field
of mind body medicine.

Chapter 2

Deepak Chopra

THE INTERVIEW

David E. Wright (Wright)
Today we are talking with Dr. Deepak Chopra, founder of the Chopra Center for Well Being in La Hoya, California. More than a decade ago, Dr. Chopra became the foremost pioneer in integrated medicine. His insights have redefined our definition of health to embrace body, mind, and spirit. His books, which include, *Quantum Healing, Perfect Health, Ageless Body Timeless Mind*, and *The Seven Spiritual Laws of Success,* have become international best sellers and established classics of their kind. His latest book is titled, *Grow Younger, Live Longer: 10 Steps to Reverse Aging.* Dr. Chopra, welcome to *A Healthier You.*

Dr. Deepak Chopra (Chopra)
Thank you. How are you?

Wright
Doing just fine. It's great weather here in Tennessee.

Chopra
Great.

Wright

Dr. Chopra, you stated in your new book that it is possible to reset your biostats up to fifteen years younger than your chronological age. Is that really possible?

Chopra

Yes. By now, we have several examples of this. The literature on aging really began to become interesting in the 1980s when it was proven possible to reverse the biological marks of aging. This included things like blood pressure, bone density, body temperature, regulation of the metabolic rate, cardiovascular conditioning, cholesterol levels, muscles mass and strength of muscles, and even things like hearing, vision, sex hormone levels, and immune function. One of the things that came out of those studies was that psychological age had a great influence on biological age. So you have three kinds of aging: chronological age is when you were born, biological age is what your biomarker shows, and psychological age is what your biostat says.

Wright

You call our prior conditioning a prison. What do you mean?

Chopra

We have certain expectations about the aging process. Women expect to become menopausal in their early forties. Everyone thinks they should retire at the age of sixty-five and then go Florida and spend the rest of their life in so-called "retirement." These expectations actually influence the very biology of aging. What we call "normal aging" is actually the hypnosis of our social conditioning. If you can bypass that social conditioning, then you're free to reset your own biological clock.

Wright

Everyone told me that I was suppose to retire at sixty-five. I'm sixty-three and, as a matter of fact, today is my birthday.

Chopra

Well happy birthday. You know, the fact is, you should be having fun *all* the time and *always* feel youthful. You should always feel that you are contributing to society. It's not the retirement per se, but it's the passion with which you're involved in the well being of your society, your community, or the world at large.

Wright

Great things keep happening to me. I have a forty-year-old daughter, but I also have a thirteen-year-old daughter. She was born when I was fifty. That has changed my life quite a bit. I feel a lot younger than I am.

Chopra

The more you associate with young people, the more you will respond to that biological expression.

Wright

Dr. Chopra, you suggest viewing our bodies from the perspective of quantum physics. That seems somewhat technical. Will you tell us a little bit more about that?

Chopra

You see, on one level, your body is made up of flesh and bone. That's the material level; but we know today that everything we consider matter is born of energy and information. By starting to think of our bodies as networks of energy, information, and even intelligence, we begin to shift our perspective. We won't think of our bodies so much as dense matter, but as vibrations of consciousness. Even though it sounds technical, everyone has had an experience with this so-called quantum body. When, for example, you do an intense workout, after the workout you feel a sense of energy in your body—a tingling sensation—you're actually experiencing what ancient wisdom traditions call the "vital force." The more you pay attention to this vital force inside your body, the more you will experience it as energy, information, and intelligence, and the more control you will have over its expressions.

Wright

Does DNA have anything to do with that?

Chopra

DNA is the source of everything in our body. DNA is the language that creates the molecules of our bodies. DNA is a protein-making factory, but DNA doesn't give us the blueprint. When I build a house, I have to go to the factory to find the bricks, but having the bricks is not enough—I need to get an architect who, in his or her consciousness can create that blueprint. That blueprint exists only in your spirit and in consciousness—in your soul.

Wright

I was interested in a statement from your last book. You said, "Perceptions create reality." What perceptions must we change in order to reverse our biological image?

Chopra

You have to change three perceptions: First you have to get rid of the perceptions of aging itself. Most people believe that aging means disease and infirmities. You have to change that. You have to regard aging as an opportunity for personal growth and spiritual growth. You also have to regard it as an opportunity to express the wisdom of your experience and an opportunity to help others and lift them from their ordinary and mundane experience to the kind of experiences you are capable of because you have much more experience than they have.

The second thing you have to do is change your perception of your physical body. You have to start to experience it as information and energy—as a network of information and intelligence.

The third thing you have to change your perception on is the experience of dying. If you are the kind of person who constantly is running out of time, then you will run out of time. On the other hand, if you have a lot of time, and if you do everything with gusto and love and passion, then you will lose track of time. And when you loose track of time, your body does not metabolize that experience.

Wright

That is interesting. People who teach time management don't really teach the passion?

Chopra

No, time management is such a restriction of time. Your biological clock starts to age much more rapidly. I think what you have to really do is live your life with passion so time doesn't mean anything to you.

Wright

That's a concept I've never heard.

Chopra

Well, there you are.

Wright

You spend an entire chapter of your book on deep rest as an important part of the reverse aging process. What is "deep rest"?

Chopra

One of the most important mechanisms for renewal and survival is sleep. If you deprive an animal of sleep, it ages very fast and dies prematurely. We live in a culture where most of our population has to resort to sleeping pills and tranquilizers to go asleep. That doesn't bring natural rejuvenation and renewal. You will know you have had a good night's sleep when you wake up in the morning and feel renewed, invigorated, and refreshed like a baby does. So that's one kind of deep rest that comes from deep sleep and from natural sleep. In the book I talk about how you make sure you get that.

The second deep rest comes from the experience of meditation, which is the ability to quiet your mind so you still your internal dialogue. When your internal dialogue is still, then you enter into a stage of deep rest; when your mind is agitated, your body is unable to rest.

Wright

You know, I have always heard of people who had bad eyesight and really didn't realize it until they went to the doctor and were fitted for lenses. I had that same experience a couple of months ago. For several years I had never really enjoyed the deep sleep you're talking about. The doctor diagnosed me with sleep apnea. Now I sleep like a baby and it makes a tremendous difference.

Chopra

Of course it does. You now have energy and the ability to concentrate and do things.

Wright

Dr. Chopra, how much do eating habits have to do with aging? Can we change and reverse our biological age by what we eat?

Chopra

Yes, you can. One of the most important things to remember is that certain types of food actually contain anti-aging compounds. There are many chemicals that are contained in certain foods that have an anti-aging effect. Most of these chemicals are derived from light. There's no way to bottle these chemicals and there are no pills you can take that will give you these chemicals. They're contained in plants rich in color and they are derived from photosynthesis. Anything that is yellow, green, and red or has a lot of color, such as fruits and vegetables, contain a lot of these very powerful anti-aging chemicals.

In addition, you have to be careful not to put food in your body that is dead or has no life energy. Anything that comes in a can or has a label, qualifies as dead—without life energy.

You can expose your body to six tastes: sweet, sour, salty, bitter, pungent, and astringent. Those are the codes of intelligence allowing us to access the deep intelligence of nature. Nature and what she gives to us in bounty is actually experienced through the sense of taste. In fact, the light chemicals—the anti-aging substances in food—create the six tastes.

Wright

I was talking to one of the ladies in your office and she sent me an invitation to a symposium you are having in March, in California. I was really interested. The title is "Exploring the Reality of Soul."

Chopra

Well, the symposium is going to be mediated by me, and I will conducted it, but we will have some of the world's foremost scientists, physicists, and biologists who are doing research in what is called, "non-local intelligence"—the intelligence of soul, or spirit. You could say it is the intelligence that orchestrates the activity of the universe—God—for example. Science and spirituality are now meeting together because by understanding how nature works and how the laws of nature work, we're beginning to get a glimpse of the deeper intelligence people in spiritual traditions call "divine," or "God." I think this is a wonderful time to explore spirituality through science. If anyone is interested in coming to this symposium, then they can go on our website, www.chopra.com and get the details.

Wright

She also sent me biographical information of the seven scientists who will be with you. I have never read a list of seven more noted people in their industry.

Chopra

They are. Included in that group is the director of the Max Planck Institute, in Berlin, Germany, where quantum physics was discovered. We will have a guest who will talk about the quantum creativity of death and the survival of conscious after death. It's an extraordinary group of people.

Wright

I think one was Hans-Peter Dürr, nuclear physicist and philosopher. The symposium sounds as if it's going to be really great. Is it a two-day event?

Chopra

Well, actually the first day is an evening reception, so it's only one day.

Wright

Dr. Chopra, with *A Healthier You*, we're trying to encourage people to be better, live better, and be more fulfilled by listening to the examples of our guest. Is there anything or anyone in your life who has made a difference for you and has helped you to become a better person?

Chopra

Well, I have to be honest; the most important person in my life was my father. Every day he said, "What can I do in thought, word, and deed to nurture every relationship I encounter just for today." That has lived with me for my entire life.

Wright

What do you think makes up a great mentor? Are there characteristics mentors seem to have in common?

Chopra

I think the most important attribute of a great mentor is that they teach by example and not necessarily through words.

Wright

When you consider the choices you've made down through the years, has faith played an important role?

Chopra

I think more than faith, what has played an important role in the choices I've made is curiosity, wonder, a sense of reverence and humility. Now, if you want to call that faith, then, yes it has.

Wright

In a divine being?

Chopra

In a greater intelligence—an intelligence who is supreme, infinite, unbounded, and too mysterious for the finite mind to comprehend.

Wright

If you could have a platform and tell our audience something you believe would help them and encourage them what would you say?

Chopra

I would say there are so many techniques that come to us from ancient wisdom and tradition that will allow us to tap into our inner resources to become beings who have intuition, creativity, vision, and a connection to that which is sacred. In finding that within ourselves, we have the means to enhance our well-being. Whether it's physical, emotional, or environmental, we have the means to resolve conflicts and get rid of war. We have the means to be really healthy. We have the means for economic uplift that says knowledge is the most important thing that exists.

Wright

I have seen you on several prime time television shows down through the years where you have had the time to explain theories and beliefs. How does a person such as I am experience this? Do we get it out of books?

Chopra

Books are tools offering a road map. But the best way is sit down every day, close your eyes and put your attention in your heart. Ask yourself two questions: who am I and what do I want? Then maintain a short period of stillness in body and mind as in prayer or meditation and the door will open for you.

Wright

So, you think that the intelligence comes from within. Do all of us have that capacity?

Chopra

Every child that is born has that capacity.

Wright

That's fascinating. So, it doesn't take trickery or anything like that?

Chopra

No, it says in the Bible in Psalms, "Be still and know that I am God."—Psalm 46:10.

Wright

That's great advice. I really do appreciate you being with us today. You are fascinating. I wish I could talk to you for the rest of the afternoon; I'm certain I am one of millions who would like to do that!

Chopra

Thank you, sir. It was a pleasure to talk with you!

Wright

Today we have been talking to Dr. Deepak Chopra founder of the Chopra Center for Well Being. More than a decade ago, he became the foremost pioneer in integrated medicine. We have found today that he really knows what he's talking about. After reading his book *Grow Younger, Live Longer, Ten Steps to Reverse Aging,* I certainly hope you'll go out to your favorite bookstore and buy a copy. Dr. Chopra, thank you so much for being with us today.

Chopra

Thank you for having me, David.

About The Author

Dr. Deepak Chopra

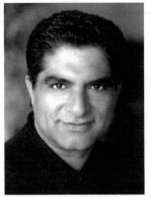

Acknowledged as one of the world's greatest leaders in the field of mind body medicine, Deepak Chopra, M.D. continues to transform our understanding of the meaning of health. Through his creation of The Chopra Center for Well Being in California in 1995, Dr. Chopra established a formal vehicle for the expansion of his healing approach using the integration of the best of western medicine with natural healing traditions. Dr. Chopra serves as the Director of Education at The Chopra Center, which offers training programs in mind body medicine (Journey into Healing). The University of California, San Diego School of Medicine has granted continuing medical education credits for this program, which satisfies requirements for the American Medical Association Physician's Recognition Award. Through his partnership with David Simon, M.D. and numerous health care professionals in both conventional and complementary healing arts, Chopra's work is changing the way the world views physical, mental, emotional, spiritual, and social wellness.

Dr. Deepak Chopra
www.chopra.com

$$Chapter\ 3$$

The Real Cure for Disabling Lower Back Injuries

Richard W. Bunch,
Ph.D., P.T., C.B.E.S.

Introduction

Unfortunately, almost everybody faces low back pain in his or her lifetime. Too often, back injuries lead to permanent disability and chronic pain. As a matter of fact, when I address middle aged or older audiences about how to prevent disabling back injuries, I inform them upfront that there two types of people present in the room, those who have back problems and know it, and those who have back problems and don't know it. This is how prevalent back problems are today, especially in the aging baby-boomer population.

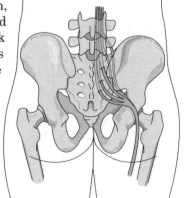

Understanding why back problems are so prevalent in modern society is essential to properly treating this condition. Proper treatment is critical because we now live in an era of fast-paced medicine where symptoms are usually treated rather than the causes. This approach leads to far too many back surgeries being performed that can easily be avoided.

The number of people in the United States who become disabled from low back injuries is growing astronomically and the truth of the matter is that much of this dilemma can be easily corrected.

First of all, let's get one thing straight—almost all back disorders are preventable. Think about it! What virus or germ causes a disc to herniate, a joint to deteriorate, or bone spur to develop in the back? The answer, of course, is none. The cause of the vast majority of neck and back disorders today is mechanical damage to the spine related to poor ergonomics—work environments that require poor postures, excessive material handling, highly repetitive motions, etc., and poor lifestyle—obesity and declining physical fitness with loss of flexibility and weakening muscle support of the neck and lower back. If a person understands how to prevent these problems by improving ergonomics and lifestyle habits, one can avoid a lot of misery from pain and complications secondary to back surgeries.

Since most back injuries result from mechanical damage, treatment can be effective if methods are used to reduce and/or reverse mechanical stresses on the damaged tissue during rehabilitation. This requires knowledge of biomechanics—the science of joint motions and reactions to internal and external forces on the body. Thus, this book chapter will address two main methodologies that provide real cures for back injuries:

 a. Ergonomics and Behavioral (Lifestyle) Changes – represents the best cure!

 b. The McKenzie method – A diagnostic-specific treatment based on the science of spinal biomechanics.

The Impact of Back Pain Today

Before describing methods of back injury treatment we need to understand the current state of affairs as it now exists in the traditional medical model for treatment of back and neck disorders. Too many people simply deal with back problems as they do with most other health issues—they do not worry about their backs until a problem occurs. Unfortunately, I have seen the impact of back injuries on the lives of numerous patients throughout the years. A ruptured disc pressing on a nerve in the lower back can cause radiating pain in the leg so severe that the person is unable to tolerate standing or sitting. When back pain prevents normal life activities such as working, driving a car, enjoying intimacy with a spouse, and caring for children, disability becomes so profound that it causes a complete deterioration of the quality of life.

Take for example a patient, John, who came to see me after undergoing five back surgeries with fusions in the period of three years without pain relief. The surgeries had failed to relieve his pain. In fact, he reported that his pain was worse than ever. Consequently, he became addicted to narcotics. He became obese, gaining more than 100 pounds because food became his only source of pleasure, and simple exercise such as walking was too painful to perform. In addition, pain medications made him feel drowsy and lethargic most of each day. He also became an alcoholic. He was consistently depressed and irritable. His personality changed so drastically as a result of depression and anger related to chronic back pain, depression, drug dependency, and alcoholism, that his wife divorced him and his children avoided him. His life was in shambles and he stated that he often thought of committing suicide. Tragically, this patient was only twenty-three years old!

I'll never forget John. He was a pipe fitter. A hard-working young man with relatively little education and who depended on physical skills to make a living. Yet, I found out that not one healthcare provider who had treated his back condition had ever once bothered to ask him about the physical demands of his job and educate him about how to take care of his back while at work and at home. This, I thought, was a form of malpractice.

As most patients today, John had received the traditional medical treatment—drugs, hot packs, massage, electrical stimulation, spinal manipulations, and spinal injections. When these methods failed to relieve pain, he finally underwent multiple back surgeries that, in turn, also failed due to complications and scar tissue formation. Consequently, the failed back surgeries made his condition worse and his disability permanent. All this at the ripe old age of twenty-three!

The failure of John's treatment program was not related to the skill of the clinicians. It was related to the fact that these treatments were directed at symptoms and not the cause. Certainly, there is a place for these treatments in medical care to help relieve pain, but they must be integrated with a diagnostic-specific approach that addresses the cause of the problem.

If poor lifestyle (e.g., lack of physical fitness) and the way we work (or ergonomics) is the primary cause of spinal injuries, then why are these methods not integral to treatment rendered by most healthcare providers today? It's extraordinarily rare when a patient says, "Oh, yes, before I went back to work after I injured my back, my doctor [or therapist] taught me proper body mechanics when handling materials, ergonomic methods to relieve stress on my spine, and posture relief exercises to keep my back healthy." Instead, the typical back patient will too often go to a healthcare provider's office, wait two hours, be seen for a few minutes and then walk out with a standard prescription for anti-inflammatory, pain medications, and/or muscle relaxants.

Understanding Back Injuries

The human spine has thirty-three bones in it called vertebrae (singular: vertebra) and in between the vertebrae are shock absorbers called discs. The disc is like a container with a very tough outer wall made of tough connective tissue, mainly collagen, that surrounds an inner core of softer material made of protein and water, often referred to as the "jelly" of the disc. In an overly simplistic view, one may look at the spinal disc as a very tough jelly doughnut.

One of the main objectives of preventing back disorders is to protect the jelly in each disc so that the shock absorption function of these structures continues to exist as we age. This is not as easy as it may seem when one understands that the average human being bends and twists the spine over 2000 times a day and exposes the lower back (lumbar) discs to hundreds of pounds of pressure when conducting common tasks such as lifting or pushing or pulling.

As mentioned, the wall of the spinal disc is made primarily of layers of collagen, the same connective tissue found in ligaments of the ankle and other joints. Since a ligament, made primarily of collagen, will heal after a sprain or tear by taking weight off the sprain by walking on crutches during the healing stage, then why will a spinal disc act any differently? The answer is that they do not. We just have a much more difficult time taking weight or pressure off the disc while it heals. If we can use a technique that relieves pressure on the disc to allow the collagen to heal, then discs should heal as easily as a sprained ankle. This technique *does* exist and will be addressed later in this chapter!

There are about twenty to thirty layers of collagen in the disc wall that are criss-crossed like the threads of a nylon tire. The criss-crossed pattern of collagen fibers in the disc wall endows the disc with tremendous strength to resist vertical compression forces. As a result, it is very hard to rupture a healthy disc.

So, why are we seeing more occurrences of degenerative disc disease and ruptured discs than ever before in our society? The answer is simple. The activities of modern life deprive the disc of nutrition and weaken the disc wall.

I first found out how this actually happens when I was in medical school studying for my doctorate in human anatomy. I learned during this time that the human disc starts to lose its blood supply at around ten years of age and by age twenty or so, the spinal discs—except for the outer wall layers—are essentially devoid of blood supply! As most people know, tissues in the body need blood supply to bring oxygen and nutrients to keep it healthy. Therefore, I was confused when I heard this information and questioned my professor as to how we can possibly keep our discs healthy if we have no blood supply after age twenty. I found out that that the discs receive nutrients from absorbing surrounding body fluids through a process called "passive osmosis." This simply means that fluids move into the disc when disc pressure is lower than the pressure of surrounding body tissues, and moves out of the disc when the disc pressure is higher than the pressure of surrounding tissues. Therefore, a healthy exchange of body fluids and waste products requires pressure in the disc to be alternatively increased and decreased over time. This occurs with dynamic movement of the spine when stretching or walking.

Sustained high disc pressures will prevent fluid uptake in the disc and therefore prohibit proper nutrition of the disc. The result is cell death in the disc that leads to weakening of the cellular structure of the disc wall, fissures (or tears) in the disc wall, disc ruptures, and disc degeneration. Certain postures such as bending forward at the waist (flexion) or sitting, increases disc pressure and prevents proper disc nutrition if sustained. Therefore, humans are not designed to be bent over a worktable or sit behind a desk all day without periodically moving the back in a way that reduces disc pressure. If we do so, we are destined suffer from disc deterioration, especially in the lower back where most pressure from spinal flexion is exerted.

Studies show that the best way to reduce disc pressure is to lie down. However, laying down while on the job is not something that employers care to advocate. Standing fully erect with good posture creates less disc pressure in the lower back than when bending forward or while sitting. Walking creates a pelvic rocking motion that helps to facilitate fluid transport in the disc, and is therefore, a healthy exercise for the lumbar spine. However, prolonged sitting has proven to be one of the big risk factors for injuring the discs in the lumbar spine. Some studies have shown that lumbar disc pressure is almost three times greater when a person sits slumped in a chair than when standing with good posture. Thus, posture and intermittent body movements are important to the health of the lumbar spine.

We now know that it is detrimental to the low back to have humans work in a bent over position as occurs when working at a welding table, a manufacturing table, or a conveyor belt. The stress on the lower back results from the upper body weight that equals about fifty-two to fifty-three percent of one's total body weight. This weight will significantly elevate the pressure in the spinal discs of the lower back (also known as the lumbar discs). Elevating lumbar disc pressure while being bent over will prevent fluid uptake in the disc much as described when sitting, and will cause the disc to deteriorate over time. Working bent forward at the waist and sitting both cause flexion of the lumbar spine.

Flexion of the lumbar spine causes wedging of the front of the disc between the vertebrae above and below. This wedging effect causes the inner disc jelly to move backwards towards the spinal nerve roots under significant internal pressure. It is the prolonged flexion of the disc or sudden overloading of the disc while in flexion that that leads to the jelly breaking through the back wall of the disc, a condition know as disc herniation.

The Effect of Common Work Postures

The effect of posture on the lumbar spine is extremely important. So what is the best posture to be in to avoid back injury? The best posture is the next posture! This means that no posture is perfect if it is maintained too long. That being said, the best static, or fixed, posture is the neutral posture. The neutral posture exists when the person sits or stands in an erect position without slumping or twisting the upper body. It is the position when the entire spine is shaped like an elongated "S" with slight inward curves of the spinal regions in the neck (cervical spine) and lower back (lumbar spine). The inward curve of the cervical and lumbar spinal areas are referred to in the medical field as "lordosis." The neutral posture of the spine is a posture that is most likely to facilitate proper fluid exchange in the spinal discs. Therefore, neutral postures in work environments, whether standing or sitting, should always be promoted. For optimum spinal health, a person should be moving out of one posture into another as often as possible. Unfortunately, many jobs today do not encourage that behavior.

The effect of prolonged sitting represents one of the most prevalent risk factors for lower back injury today. An office worker, for example, sits most of the day, commutes seated in a car, and too often sits at home while watching television for hours while recovering from the stresses of the day.

A truck driver represents the worse example of all for lumbar injuries. A truck driver sits all day long and is exposed to seated whole body vibration from the moving vehicle. Seated vibration is harmful to the spine as it causes fluid to be pushed out of the disc at a higher rate than when sitting without exposure to vibration. Thus, vibration can cause the disc to dehydrate and degenerate at higher than normal rates. To make matters worse, truck drivers also lift when loading and unloading the trucks. Thus, truck drivers are exposed to a triple whammy—prolonged seated postures, vibration exposures, and high compressive forces from lifting. Incidentally, truck drivers experience the highest rates of back injuries in the country.

Research also shows that the same mechanism of lower back injury from exposure to seated vibration also affects the average person who drives a car each day. In fact, studies have shown that people who drive automobiles for more than two hours per day (i.e., while commuting) have three times the risk of experiencing a herniated disc in the lumbar spine than people who do not.

It is just a common physiological fact. Prolonged sitting and forward bending of the trunk while standing leads to fluid being pushed out of the disc and prohibits fluid exchange. With no blood supply to replace the fluid you lose, unless you stand straight and move your spine as when walking, body fluids can not move into the disc to bring the fresh nutrients and oxygen it needs to keep that inner jelly healthy and that collagen healthy. Consequently, unless a person moves periodically the disc has no choice but to degenerate over time or even herniate, and cause pain.

To make matters worse, there is often no early warning system that can alert you when spinal discs become injured or begin to herniate. For all practical purposes, spinal discs have no pain receptors in the jelly core and inner two thirds of the wall of the disc. There is only a sparse number of pain receptors located in the outer one third of the disc wall. This means that discs often herniate well before any pain is perceived. Therefore, disc herniation, for the most part, is a silent process. This explains why scientific studies reveal that MRIs will show herniated discs in about one third of non-symptomatic (pain-free) adults older than age thirty.

This also explains how a person can experience sudden pain from a herniated disc upon performing a simple task such as bending over to tie a shoelace. The actual event of tying the shoelace did not herniate the disc. The disc was already herniated but not painful prior to this simple task. Bending over simply was the last straw that led to herniation of the disc to the point that pain fibers in the outer one third of the wall were activated.

In some cases, a herniated disc will bulge out far enough to press directly on a nerve root and cause severe, excruciating extremity pain and numbness. Therefore, poor postures that increase disc pressures for prolonged periods of time and material handling that increases disc pressure to such high levels as to cause tears in the disc can result in a process called "cumulative trauma." This term applies very aptly to the spine because trauma accumulates in the disc and the other tissues of the body well before we are aware of it.

Like prolonged sitting, prolonged standing can cause lower back pain. However, the joints in the spine behind the discs, called the "facet joints," and not the spinal discs themselves, typically cause lower back pain in response to prolonged standing. Each typical vertebra has four facet joints, two upper and two lower. Unlike spinal discs, facet joints are very pain sensitive. During prolonged standing the abdominal muscles begin to relax and this allows the pelvis to tilt downward. The downward tilt of the pelvis causes the lumbar spine to move into excessive lordosis (i.e., excessive curvature) as seen when a person exhibits a sway-backed posture. The result is excessive mechanical compression of the lumbar facet joints and related pain.

Pregnant women can relate to lower back pain, especially during the third trimester when the swayed-back posture is most prominent. As an ergonomic consultant for a casino, I became aware of card dealers' complaints of lower back pain while stand-

ing. Anybody who has ever experienced lower back pain from prolonged standing has found that back
pain can be relieved by placing one
foot up on a stool or other object.
The pain relief resulted from the
pelvis tilting backwards and
straightening out the excessively
curved lumbar spine as the hip is
flexed to lift the foot. Reducing an
excessively curved lumbar spine
reduces pressure on the facet joints
and thereby reduces joint compression pain. In the casinos where I
have consulted I recommended placing short step stools under the
gaming tables to allow the dealers to lift one foot up and relieve
facet joint pressure on the lumbar spine. Simple ergonomic
changes like this can prevent back pain and unnecessary medical
treatment.

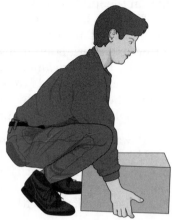

Back Injuries and Lifting

Eighty-three percent of all lifting injuries occur in the bent
over posture, usually with the legs straight, bending from the
waist. Many people have heard, "Bend your legs when you lift,"
but they really don't understand why. When a person bends over
with the legs straight to lift an object, the pressure in the discs
from the weight of the upper body combined with the weight of
the object being lifted becomes phenomenal. If you lift a fifty-
pound object, studies show that in the first one second of the lift
you will generate more than 1,250 pounds of disc pressure in your
lower lumbar spine!

As previously mentioned, one of the leading causes of disc herniation, is bending forward or flexing the lower back. This is
especially true when lifting. However, twisting the upper body
while flexing the spine is even more stressful and damaging to
the disc and surrounding tissues of the back. For maximum damage to the spine one only has to bend and twist the upper back
while lifting something. If the lift occurs with the hands held
away from the body, sudden back injury can occur even when lifting relatively light objects due to the magnification effect from
increasing the lever arm. The golden rule of lifting therefore is to

keep the load close to the body when lifting to minimize the pressure in the lumbar spine.

The first line of defense against back injuries from lifting is for employers to try as best as they can to engineer out manual lifting of materials by using hoists, cranes, conveyor belts, forklifts, etc. If lifting cannot be engineered out of a job, then proper lifting technique needs to be strictly adhered to. When manually lifting, the load must always be kept close to the body and a person should follow the B.L.A.S.T. technique. B.L.A.S.T. stands for:

B – Bow the back in (keep the normal inward curve)
L – Use the legs to lift, not the back
A – Abdominal muscles: Tighten them to stabilize the lumbar spine S – Slow and smooth: Never jerk while lifting
T – Twisting: Never do it!

Effect of Lifestyle on Lower Back Injuries

Sedentary lifestyles contribute to obesity that in turn causes extra weight to be borne on the spinal discs. Obesity has become a national epidemic with approximately two-thirds of adults being overweight or obese. For every extra pound of weight in the upper body, there is an estimated increase of four pounds of lumbar disc pressure. Therefore, a person carrying fifty pounds of excess upper body weight will, on average, increase lumbar disc pressure by approximately 200 pounds!

Declining physical fitness often results in weakening of the abdominal and back muscles. These muscles are critical to protecting the lumbar spine, especially when lifting. Weakness of the abdominal and back muscles leads to poor support of the lower back and further deterioration of the spine.

Consider that the peak times in life for serious disc herniations requiring surgery is anywhere from thirty-five years of age to about fifty years old. This time period corresponds to when people are still working but have become deconditioned from lack of physical activity. Despite the declining physical fitness levels of employees, physical demands of a job may not change and consequently expose employees to greater physical stress.

After consulting and being cleared by their medical physicians, it is strongly recommended that people perform aerobic exercises and eat properly to lose weight. Eating properly means cutting down total caloric intake, avoiding high glycemic foods, and foods high in saturated and trans fats.

To burn calories and improve cardiovascular fitness, aerobic exercise should be conducted at least forty-five minutes every day. This can involve simply walking at a quick pace to increase heart rate and energy expenditure. We need to burn more calories than we ingest in order to lose excessive weight. In addition, people should perform modified sit-ups called crunches and push-ups to strengthen the abdominal and chest muscles.

Other strengthening exercises for the arms and legs are strongly encouraged. Flexibility of the back should be maintained by stretching every day. These are healthy lifestyle recommendations that will provide benefits that extend beyond back injury prevention. They will also help reduce life threatening cardiovascular problems and other diseases.

Curing Back Injuries by Prevention

It is apparent that lower back injuries occur both with sedentary jobs and physically demanding jobs. The mechanisms of back injury just differ. In sedentary jobs, the typical back problem results from weakening of discs and associated tissues from poor, prolonged sitting postures and a lack of spinal motion. In other words, sedentary work deprives the discs of nutrition from lack of movement.

In physically demanding jobs, the mechanism of injury typically involves awkward, prolonged, bent-over postures and stresses from lifting. These causes of back problems are well known and documented in the medical literature. So why do we continue with "shake and bake" physical therapy treatments using only passive modalities such as heat and electrical stimulation, massage, chiropractic manipulations, drugs, and injections? Do any of these techniques actually reverse the tissue damage and cause a disc bulge to be reduced? These techniques do not teach people how to avoid repeating the mechanical irritation of the spine at work and home. So, why are these traditional methods so often used as the primary or only treatments for back injures today? Can ineffective therapies be the cause of unnecessary back surgeries? Considering that back surgeries often have complications, mainly from scar tissue, we need to give serious consideration as to how we are treating back injuries today. So, let's discuss the *real* cure for most back injuries.

First, everyone who sits throughout the day in a car, truck, crane, or office needs to understand how crucial it is to avoid prolonged sitting without using a lumbar support cushion and without getting up periodically to move. In office environments, a good ergonomic chair that is adjusted properly for the body is indispensable. A lumbar cushion positioned in the lower back region will help maintain the spine in its normal curvature and promote tissue fluid transport that is so necessary for the health of the avascular disc. Otherwise, sitting with the lower back flattened as occurs when sitting slumped, will flex the spine, compress the discs, prohibit fluid transport into the disc and prevent proper disc nutrition. Crossing the legs or sitting on one leg while working at computer stations also flattens the lower back, increases lumbar disc pressure, and prohibits disc nutrition. These behaviors, therefore, should be strongly discouraged. Getting up from the seated position to stretch at least every thirty minutes, even if only for a few seconds, has proven to be a great method to improve disc nutrition and prevent lower back problems.

When standing for prolonged periods in one location on a job, try to have a railing or small step stool positioned so that one foot can be propped up and supported to flex the hip and help maintain the normal alignment of the spine. Switch between propping the right and left foot throughout the day. A person who stands most of the time at work should try to occasionally sit to relieve the fatigue of standing. Sit/lean chairs provide an alternative that allows fatigue relief characteristic of sitting while at the same time allowing reduced lumbar disc pressure characteristic of standing. It is important to wear good shoes with proper arch supports and use anti-fatigue mats at work to help reduce the stress on the lower back (and arches of the feet) from prolonged standing.

We need to periodically stretch throughout the day to promote fluid transport in the spinal discs and in the joints of our body. The physiological necessity for movement to maintain health has never changed among human beings throughout time. We are designed to move! We were meant to run through the jungles, chase furry animals, and squat by the fireplace! Instead we find ourselves sitting or standing in one position all day, glued to computers, driving cars to go everywhere rather than walk, and taking escalators and elevators rather than take the stairs. It seems that human beings today almost go out of their way to avoid moving!

Richard W. Bunch,
Ph.D., P.T., C.B.E.S.

A smart way to help combat sedentary jobs and lifestyles is to integrate exercise with work. Simple activities such walking up and down stairs rather than taking elevators, and parking the car far way from the office building so that walking is required are excellent ways to increase activity levels, move the spine, and burn more calories.

Stretching daily is essential to the health of the spine and other joints in the body. A very successful stretching program that I designed for many industries is called the "WUPR" program. WUPR stands for warm-up, and posture relief. The method is really simple. For instance, if there is a lot of bending over at the waist while standing involved in job tasks, then people should warm up before working by doing standing toe-touch stretching exercises that will gently stretch the lower back. This technique can help prevent unnecessary lower back sprains and strains. Unlike warm-up exercises that prepare the body's tissues to withstand stress before the job is initiated, posture relief exercises are performed during and after the job to relieve or repair tissue damage from activities that involve stressful postures. In other words, posture relief exercises are exercises that counter the harmful effect of bad postures. Performing back extensions, for example, after being bent over is a key posture relief exercise.

Standing back extension as a posture relief exercise deserves special recognition. Back extensions have been shown to reduce disc pressure in the lower back and move the jelly in the disc forward away from the back wall of the disc. In other words, it does everything to help prevent the disc from herniating! This is a particularly important posture relief exercise to be done every thirty minutes by office workers. On the other hand, back extensions would not typically be posture relief exercises for people who stand all day. Since standing promotes the swayed back posture and places the lumbar spine in relative extension, back flexion exercises such as standing toe-touches would then become the posture relief exercise of choice. Therefore, whether an exercise is considered a "warm-up" or "posture relief" exercise depends on the specific circumstances and postures being addressed. Side bends and back rotations can be warm-up stretches for tasks that require these motions or can be posture relief exercise to counter these motions. This simple approach of WUPR has helped many of my industry clients reduce back injuries by more than sixty-three percent on average! Think of the suffering, medical costs, lost work time, reduced productivity, and potential disability this simple approach has eliminated!

Ergonomic changes in the work environment have become a big issue today because of escalating musculoskeletal injuries like back injuries. In the ergonomic training courses I provide to industry clients, I teach that we always manage ergonomic issues with three primary objectives in mind. Engineering out a problem is the primary ergonomic objective. This concept works for the home environment as well as the work environment. For example, if I visit a person's garage I will usually find the five-gallon gasoline tank for a lawnmower that weighs about thirty-eight pounds stored on the floor. Yet, the much lighter one-pound hammer is neatly placed at waist level right on top of a tool table. A simple engineering change would be to have the five-gallon gasoline tank stored on a rolling cart with a siphon hose so a person would be able to avoid lifting the tank from the floor and minimize handling the heavy tank. This eliminates one risk of unnecessarily straining the lower back while lifting the gasoline tank from the floor. There are a myriad of similar engineering changes that can be conducted at work and at home that represent either no cost or low cost solutions for reducing risks of back injuries.

Administrative intervention represents the second ergonomic objective. This can involve job rotation so that an employee does not perform the same task over and over. This helps to promote changes in postures that are good for a healthy back.

The third ergonomic objective is behavioral modification. Relying on behavior is always the least reliable method for injury prevention but it cannot be neglected. Proper behaviors represent such actions as performing posture relief exercises and using proper body mechanics during lifting.

The overall goal of any ergonomic program is to eliminate or reduce excessive force, awkward postures, and excessive repetitive motions. In addition, reducing exposures of the body to whole body vibration and extremes of heat and cold are also methods to help reduce the incidences of back injuries and other health problems.

Prevention after all, is always the best cure as once stated by the venerable Benjamin Franklin. Yet in the United States we spend much more money on reactive treatment of problems rather than proactive approaches involving preventative measures. Ergonomics and behavioral-based safety, in my opinion, is more effective in preventing lower back injuries than any medical treatment that exists today.

Curing Back Injuries by Diagnostic-Specific Non-Invasive Treatment — The McKenzie approach

Let's face it, despite all our best efforts we may still end up having a back injury. What will a person do when back pain is severe or leg pain develops from a compressed spinal nerve? Who should a person see and what type of treatment will really work?

There exists today a specialized, highly effective spinal evaluation and treatment program called the "McKenzie" spinal assessment. The McKenzie approach is a biomechanical method of spinal evaluation that will identify a specific treatment regime that empowers the patient to repair the disc and restore function without dependency on the clinician. This approach really appealed to me when I first heard the originator, Robin McKenzie, a physical therapist from New Zealand, present his technique during a medical conference. The concept involves developing a specific exercise pattern that affects the spine in such a way as to relieve the pressure on a spinal nerve, reduce pressure on the damaged disc wall, regain disc integrity, and most importantly restore the person to full, pain-free function again. The patient is given information on what to at home and what to avoid doing. Once instructed on these issues, the patient is fully expected to comply and take full responsibility for his or her recovery. Rather than being brought into the clinic every day the patient is told to come in on periodic intervals to reassess progress and to make changes in the program as needed. I commonly treat herniated discs with nerve root pain successfully using the McKenzie approach, often in as little as three sessions, even when patients have been told that he or she needed back surgery!

Since I have been trained in the McKenzie method of spinal assessment and treatment I have applied this approach to back and neck patients with a remarkable success rate exceeding ninety percent! Many of my peers trained in the McKenzie technique share the same findings. It is important to know that disc herniations do not all behave alike and respond to different exercise patterns. Thus, each back patient must be individually assessed and time must be spent to identify the exercise patterns of movement that will best remedy the condition.

The McKenzie approach is one that is based on the correct concept of physical evaluation. The evaluation requires significant time to perform correctly but the results indicate that the time is well worth it. The McKenzie technique makes the patient less dependent on the clinician. Isn't this the way we should be practicing medicine today? Yet despite the consistent great results derived from this methodology, the McKenzie technique is not taught in most medical schools! This is amazing. Many medical doctors know of the technique but very few use it personally in their practices as the evaluation is too time consuming for the busy schedule of a medical doctor. There are so many other things that medical physicians must be concerned with such as life-threatening health problems, complicated illnesses and injuries that truly require surgeries. Good doctors understand that they can't be all things to all people and commonly refer back and neck patients to McKenzie-certified physical therapists, relying on them to determine whether or not the correct form of diagnostic-specific conservative intervention will work.

Obviously, this book chapter cannot do justice to describing the McKenzie technique. My purpose here was to make everyone who reads this chapter aware that such a beneficial technique does exist. It is non-invasive and empowers the patient to take charge of his or her own recovery. This is very appealing to most people with legitimate back problems.

The best way to locate a certified McKenzie physical therapist in any area of the United States or abroad is to refer to the web site www.McKenzieMDT.org. Once one has entered the web site, all one has to do is enter an address or zip code. In response, a list of McKenzie certified clinicians within the designated geographical region code will appear on the screen complete with telephone numbers and addresses. Unless an emergency back pain situation exists that is unstable or life threatening, I strongly recommend that a person consult with a McKenzie-certified licensed physical therapist as soon as back pain occurs and particularly before resorting to any elective back surgeries or other invasive treatment procedures.

Summary

Hopefully, this chapter has pointed out how a low back injury, one of the leading causes of occupational disability, can be easily prevented and treated successfully. Life is too short as it is. We do not need to shorten it further by destroying our quality of life by having disabling back pain that can be prevented or successfully treated.

Be smart and take control of your life. Learn more about ergonomics and use basic ergonomic principles as presented in this book chapter to prevent back injuries. Be a smart consumer of medicine and critically analyze any medical procedure offered to you for back pain. Always ask the basic question: How does a medical treatment truly address the cause of my problem? Consider the McKenzie method for non-invasive treatment of back and neck problems. Being smart about taking care of your back may well be one of the best decisions of your life!

About The Author

Dr. Richard Bunch, PhD, PT, CBES

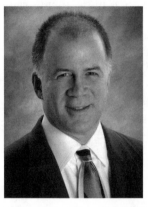 Dr. Bunch is a highly sought after nationally renown public speaker, author, and consultant on the topics of wellness and ergonomics. As a clinician, ergonomic consultant and motivational injury prevention and wellness speaker he has helped over 900,000 employees reduce their risks to musculoskeletal injuries such as neck, back, shoulder and carpal tunnel problems, improve fitness, control stress, lose weight and significantly reduce their risk of diabetes, cancer and heart disease. His training programs have directly helped industries reduce medical problems by as much as 78%. Dr. Bunch attended the U.S. Military Academy at West Point, and later became a licensed physical therapist and ergonomic specialist with a medical Ph.D. in Human Anatomy. He is a member of the National Speakers Association (NSA). As a native Louisianan, based out of new Orleans, Dr. Bunch is well noted for blending Cajun humor in his seminars with the belief that along with all the wonderful health tips he addresses, that laughter is still good medicine. He can be contacted at (800)414-2174 or by e-mail, Bunchisr@AOL.com.

Richard W. Bunch, PhD, PT, CBES
ISR Institute
1516 River Oaks Road West
New Orleans, Louisiana 70123
Phone: 800.414.2174
Phone: 504.733.2111
Fax: 504.733.5999
E-mail: Bunchisr@AOL.com
www.isr-institute.com

Chapter 4

COOL, CALM AND PRODUCTIVE

Lynn Shaw, MSW

Imagine enjoying a full twenty-four hours doing something you enjoy, appreciating the challenges of the activity, and then returning to the same experience twenty-four hours later. As you visualize this, would any of it be related to...work?

I relish the end of a workday whether it's at 5 P.M. or 5 A.M. I look forward to something else. But sometimes when I arrive at what I thought was going to be my "fun time," I find I'm not as energetic as when I began my drive home. Maybe I don't want to open mail, fix a meal, or meet with friends. Maybe I just want to flip on the television. Maybe I just want to go to bed.

Being cool, calm, and productive is more than flipping a switch inside you from home to work and from work to home. It is an intentional commitment to bring your best to wherever you are.

My background in psychotherapy has given me a rich and diverse perspective on how to generate a daily existence of remaining cool, choosing calm, and staying on task. Most of my work has been in the arena of stress and change and its impact on our emotional and mental beings. As part of my training during the past decade, I found the concepts of therapeutic laughter to be a wonderful adjunct to my traditional psychotherapy practice. I came up with a solid model I call, "Workin' the TEE HEE," by drawing from the experiences of the hundreds of patients and clients I've been privileged to know then contemplating my own overhaul of how I choose to live. Each letter of the words, TEE HEE represents the six elements of the formula—the six components to practice every day for a life of wholeness and wellness:

T – Time
E – Enthusiasm
E—Energy
H—Health
E—Encouragement
E—Exercise

As you review the TEE HEE, you will find a description for each component. At the end of this description, you will have the opportunity to explore a question and then take action. The action is in the form of a commitment task to move you into a plan of wellness for your mind, body, and spirit. You will readily recognize that the six components are a reminder of what you say you will do or want to do, and by committing to a focused action, you will be Workin' the TEE HEE! It's your turn to claim the energy, passion, and purpose to live each day being cool, calm, and productive. Ready? Let's move and get workin'!

T – TIME

Time management experts ask us to prioritize, delegate, and become former procrastinators in order to effectively use our time. Multi-tasking has become a household concept as we cram as much movement into each minute as possible. You've seen multi-taskers eat, talk, run, read, laugh, look, and listen all at once!

In the past week, have you taken time to:
- Call a friend
- Sleep more than five hours in one stretch
- Write a letter (not e-mail)
- Play with a pet
- Dream
- Clear clutter

If you answer no to any of the above, then your challenge is to see time as not just a commodity but as an opportunity. Take time during the next twenty-four hours to be purposeful about what needs to be in your life that can calm a frazzled nerve, collect a wandering thought, and produce a healthier you. Yes, I agree that showing up for work and doing your job is doing something for others. Most people I have met focus more on not having enough time rather than being purposeful about time. Have you said recently:

- "Where does the time go?"
- "There's not enough time to do it all."
- "I'm too busy to add anything else."
- "I was only going to spend fifteen minutes checking e-mail and two hours have passed!"
- *"They* just don't manage their time well."

The element of time in this formula is not about filling a palm pilot, a planner, or a fifteen-minute increment in a day's work. It is choosing to take time to replenish your spirit with a focused and specific action. An example of replenishing one's spirit is my friend, Ned. He is an eighty-one-year-old "young" man who knows how to be cool, calm, and productive with his time. He soars every day with multiple tasks. He runs from the time he gets up until the time he gets in bed. He fills his time with planning and presenting workshops for high school students at least twenty-nine out of fifty-two weekends a year. He calls friends every day and calls his three sons once a week. He reads something to edify his work and his spirit every day. He has amazed me and amused me with his energy. Does he get tired? Of course! So he takes time to rest. Then the next day, he's up with purpose and intention to create opportunities with his time.

Focus: What are you willing to do differently with your time to create a healthier you? Be intentional—do not guess. Be purposeful—be aware of what will feed your mind, body, and spirit in the next twenty-four hours you have said you would take time to do but have not.

Commit: I will commit to take time in the next twenty-four hours to:

_____.

E – ENTHUSIASM

Several years ago, managers started their teams' meetings with the question, "How's your PMA (Positive Mental Attitude)?" Teams would respond, "Boy, am I enthusiastic!" Today if you ask someone how's their PMA, they think you're referring to a palm pilot, techno-gadget, or computer software.

According to Steve Harrell, author of *Attitude is Everything*, enthusiasm is infectious, contagious, and is hugely responsible for 100 percent positive attitude.

What level of enthusiasm do you bring to your work, your home, your tasks?

On a scale of one to ten with ten being the most enthusiasm your body can wiggle, how do you measure your enthusiasm:

_____ upon rising
_____ preparing for the day
_____ arriving at work
_____ attending meetings
_____ eating
_____ childcare
_____ elder care
_____ arriving at home
_____ evening activities
_____ retiring for the night

Add up your score knowing that not each of these will fit you. You can gauge how enthusiastic you are being simply by looking at any category with less than a seven marked by it.

How do you create authentic enthusiasm?

- Be cheerfully challenged
- Be curiously committed
- Be in creative control

A study about stress resistance in executives found that after eight years of following these men and women in high stress situations, their enthusiasm was still running their companies. What made the difference in a rocky economic climate? The researcher found what she called the three C's: challenged, creative, and control. The executives focused on problems as challenges and opportunities that called for an enthusiastic response. They didn't waste any time on what they could not control so their enthusiasm targeted what they could control. They utilized creative brainstorming solution-oriented outcomes so their enthusiasm was contagious.

Focus: How's your PMA? Do you answer, "Am I enthusiastic," or, do you exclaim, "I *am* enthusiastic!"

Commit: Practice this laughter exercise to generate enthusiasm: Smile five times in five seconds, ready...one, two, three, four, five! You should feel the stretch in your smile lines and perhaps start to chuckle. You may also feel silly. Good. The word silly comes from the word "*sileas*," which translates to "blessed." So step into blessed any and every chance you get. It is infectious.

E—ENERGY

Do you say this at least once a day? "I just don't have any energy," or, "My energy is low," or "She/He has so much energy!" "If I could just bottle my child's energy!" Energy—many are talking about how to get it, how to keep it or how to give it away!

Energy is powerful. Energy runs our day because when we run out of energy we run out of power. Energy is created in a variety of ways, many of which are described in other chapters. For this section, I want you to focus on replenishing your energy.

Here are three suggestions to replenish your energy:

1. Peppermint—Researchers have concluded that peppermint can restore your energy either through a mint itself or through peppermint oil. At a workshop, I was asked to take a few drops of peppermint oil, rub it on my hands and then place one hand behind my neck and massage. I was then asked to inhale the peppermint fragrance. The tingling sensation on the back of my neck and the awakening of my smelling sensors indicated I was responding energetically to the peppermint. To this day, peppermint mints are in my house and I drink peppermint tea for a lift.

2. Tootsie Rolls—My favorite treat (low fat of course) is the fun Tootsie Roll®. I am a self-professed chocoholic. I have enjoyed the chewy challenge of a big Tootsie Roll for many years past childhood. When I was researching energy, I wanted to find one item I could give to people to represent energy. For some reason, tootsie rolls came to mind. If you go to www.tootsie.com, you will find incredible stories of how these candies provided energy for U.S. soldiers. The following is reprinted with permission by Clifford W. Meyer who served in the Korean War as a Marine corporal, and member of the Third Battalion Seventh Marine Regiment. "During November 1950 the First Marine Divi-

sion with elements of two Regimental combat teams of the U.S. Army, a Detachment of British Commandos and some South Korean Policemen—about 15,000 men—faced the Chinese Communist Army's ten Divisions totaling 120,000 men. "At a mountain reservoir called Chang Jin (we called it 'Chosin') temperatures ranged from minus five degrees below zero in the day to minus twenty-five degrees below zero at night. The ground froze so hard that bulldozers could not dig emplacements for our Artillery. The cold impeded our weapons from firing automatically, slowing down the recoil of our artillery and automatic weapons. The cold numbed our minds, froze our fingers and toes and froze our rations. [We were] seventy-eight miles from the sea, surrounded, supplies cut, facing an enemy whose sole objective was the annihilation of the First Marine Division as a warning to other United Nations troops, and written off as lost by the high command. "A war correspondent asked if we were going to retreat. The Commanding General, First Marine Division General Oliver Prince Smith replied 'Retreat? Hell, we are attacking in another direction.' "Col. Murray said 'We are coming out with our dead, our wounded and our equipment, we are coming out as Marines or we are not coming out at all.' "We put our seriously wounded in sleeping bags, and secured our dead to the fenders and hoods of the trucks. Those we had no space for we buried. Every Marine became a rifleman. Unable to build a fire to heat our rations the men were close to starvation. Destroying non-essential equipment, we discovered boxes and boxes of Tootsie Rolls, frozen solid from the sub-zero temperature. The Tootsie Rolls were issued to all the men. The sugar gave us energy and the candy satisfied our hunger. After two weeks of bitter fighting we finally reached the sea with most of our dead, our wounded, our equipment, and one very important extra: 100,000 North Korean Civilians voting for freedom with their feet following us out. Some of them live in the United States today. The 15,000 Soldiers and Marines suffered over 12,000 casualties, 3,000 killed, 6,000 wounded and thousands of frostbite cases. "Ask any man that served at the Chosin, to be good a Tootsie Roll must be frozen!"

3. Laughter—When was the last time you laughed so hard that tears ran down your legs? A good belly laugh has so many benefits we take for granted. Replenishing your energy with laughter has one requirement—a playful heart. When you access your playful heart, you open yourself to connecting with others in laughter. Connections always contain energy! Toddlers with their toothless wide-smiled grins are amazing at transforming energy. Just watching a two-year-old run and discover brings smiles to weary faces. High-pitch giggles floating down a staircase relaxes a tension-filled room. Knowing someone who snorts when they laugh helps others laugh out loud! For a moment, imagine the fragrance of peppermint in the palm of your hand. Lift your hand and inhale the aroma of strong, crisp, clean peppermint. Ahhhh. Now stretch your smile muscles as wide as they can go...and release. Smile naturally—feel the energy start to expand from your smile muscles to your eyes. Open your eyes wide and lower your jaw. You should have a wide-open smile that a laughter sound can come forth. Breathe into a ha, ha, ha and feel the energy continue to expand through your lungs as you replenish your mind, your body, and your spirit. And, just for fun, have a laughter snort! Tee Hee!

Focus: What are other ways you can replenish your energy that will access your creativity and fun?

Commitment: Today I will replenish my energy by:

_____

H—HEALTH

Throughout this book, you are being encouraged to consider how to create and maintain a healthier you for mind, body, and spirit. You will be inspired to exercise differently, meditate, or participate in yoga. You will be asked to think differently to originate a different mindset for you and your body.

Where do you live mentally? Where do you spend the majority of your waking time in your thoughts? Your mental health is as significant as the aerobic exercise you do to benefit your heart and lungs. How you think about yourself and your life will be reflected in your daily choices.

Do you live with worrisome thoughts? Do you live with angry thoughts? Do you stay in sad thinking? Do you dip into admonishing yourself for imperfections or perceived or not so perceived foolish behavior?

Sometimes our mental health needs a break as much as our physical workouts.

If you have been pushing yourself mentally to exhaustion, you know it because your brain feels fogged and you can't articulate a string of sentences in the same breath. You have been bombarded with information from all kinds of time-saving instruments and your brain has screamed, *enough!* It's time for a fresh perspective.

Your health is not just your body and your mind—it's all-consuming—it's how you breathe, think, move, sleep, eat, exercise, etc. Health is crucial to being transformed from tired to terrific. Focusing on your health daily encompasses the four previous components of TEE HEE. Take time to think about your dreams. Be creatively challenged to exercise your mind. Create energy through positive thoughts and commit to believing what you say you will do. Relax those mental hoops long enough to step over them.

One of my favorite mantras is, "This is temporary and I can handle anything in the moment." This mental exercise helps me draw my energy and resources to the full present. By bringing my mind to the present, I can regroup and refocus.

Another fun way to clear thoughts is to laugh—out loud. It is physically impossible to laugh and think at the same time. Oh, you think you're thinking when you're laughing because we laugh so quickly. Most adults sustain laughter for three to five seconds, that's it! Combine several laughter sounds together and you can increase those increments, and clear the cobwebs from your mind. The result? You attain clarity for positive mental health.

Focus: Where do I live mentally? What prevents me from having clarity?

Commitment: The mantra I create today to gain clarity for positive mental health is:

_____

E—ENCOURAGEMENT

Raise your right arm straight up in the air. Turn your palm back. Bend your elbow and pat yourself on the back three times just for being here! When was the last time you got a pat on the back?

Encouragement is the act of acknowledgment. It is recognizing when someone needs to be strengthened in spirit. Encouraging others is being aware of who is in your space.

Two weeks after 9/11, I had to fly to a speaking engagement. As I arrived at the airport and noticed the security personnel, the national guardsmen walking around in full combat attire, and the tense faces of airline personnel, I knew I was going to be very intentional about my words and my actions. A colleague had given me a button that said, "You Make a Difference." Why I had that button in my pocket that day, I do not recall. After I had checked in for my flight and having had a cordial, swift, no-nonsense exchange with the airline agent, I reached in my pocket, took out the button and passed it over to the agent. I said, "Thank you. You do make a difference." Gone was the tension from her face as her eyes widened when she read the button. She then made direct eye contact with me accompanied by a smile. "Thank you!" she exclaimed and then turned to the agent standing beside her and beamed. I walked on to my gate feeling a lot lighter than the guns the guardsmen were carrying.

Giving and receiving encouragement takes a few moments. I'm not asking you to drop your commitments and run out the door to the world on a mission to encourage. I am asking you to each day bring encouragement to your space. Whoever you encounter is someone to encourage, to lift up, to inspire, to care about, to listen to, to talk with, to be in silence with, and to instill belief.

Encouragement can begin with random acts of kindness, and it can build with daily, intentional awareness. How many times have I walked past the same crossing guard at the elementary school without a nod? How many times have I seen the same elderly man sitting alone outside the grocery store? Yes, he's known as being odd and he is harmless to humankind. Who speaks to him? How many times have you ridden the same bus with the same bus driver and just dropped your tokens in without looking at the person behind the uniform?

How many times have you listened to the same rabbi, teacher, minister, leader and dozed off listening to the familiar drone of their voice without noticing if there are any tired lines around their eyes or if their passion for their calling is being challenged?

Replenishing your spirit with encouragement is helping others to stress less and choose calm. You are productive when you offer yourself to others whether it's a quick e-mail to acknowledge someone's efforts or a phone call to make it even more personal.

It is also important for you to be replenished by receiving encouragement. Do you shrug off others' efforts to praise you? Do you toss a hand-written "thank you" as insignificant? Do you turn a shoulder to an out-reached hand? Do you forget to withdraw for alone time to replenish yourself and your energy? How open are you to receiving encouragement?

Focus: Think of one person today who needs to be encouraged. What do you see? What could you do to acknowledge them today?

Commitment: Today I will encourage (fill in the name) _____ by an act of acknowledgement, (fill in what you will do) _____.

E—EXERCISE

Therapeutic laughter as exercise is a delicious way to create A Healthier You!

In 2000, I became involved with laughter clubs through the World Laughter Tour, Inc. As a Certified Laughter Leader, I led a laughter club at our local hospital. It was amazing to hear reports from people who chose to participate. Without jokes or one-liners, we showed up and participated in thirty-minute laughter exercise programs combining yoga breathing, stretching, and silly (blessings) laughter exercises. People with depression, anxiety, worry, and tense, tired bodies would show up. People with headaches, backaches, and sore muscles participated. Afterwards, the same people reported feeling better, the headache gone, the muscle soreness relieved, and the mood shifting from dark to light. (Check out www.laughterclubs.com for information.)

Therapeutic laughter is the physical act of laughing which results in tremendous physiological and psychological benefits. Dr. Lee Berk, a researcher with Loma Linda University, reports that it only takes twenty seconds of laughter to have the same physical benefit of three minutes of rowing a boat! Talk about an aerobic activity! You do not have to get a joke, a story, or wait for laughter—you already possess all the equipment you need.

The physical scientists like Dr. Berk are catching up with us social scientists who already knew how laughter transforms lives. It's wonderful to now have data supporting our results. When I introduced therapeutic laughter in my counseling practice, it was after I had spent a week training in understanding the cathartic process of laughter and tears. I learned that simulated laughter can be just as beneficial as stimulated laughter. I asked my clients to look for laughter every day and to practice saying, "Tee Hee" after a negative thought.

This unscientific study from my practice produced interesting results. Women and men of all ages embraced the act of laughing. One man—a bank employee for twenty-six years—found the words, Tee Hee, just helped him smile. He didn't even have to say it out loud. One woman who was accustomed to using profanity under her breath toward her supervisor, switched to saying Tee Hee. Those who embraced the idea that laughter was another tool to cope with stress and change reported feeling lighter sooner than my clients who didn't.

Exercising the mind, body, and spirit with laughter also invites other types of movement. Dancing of any kind can be freeing and filled with laughter whether dancing alone or with a group. Running and feeling that "runner's high" brings smiles of achievement. Walking for fitness and leisure connects you to the fluid movement of your body one heel-to-toe step at a time. The key element of exercise is en**joy**ment. Invite the joy into your purposeful and intentional movement.

Focus: What type of exercise do you want to embrace to remain cool, choose calm, and stay productive? Whatever type of exercise you do, enjoy it and bring laughter to it.

Commitment: Today I will laugh out loud at least _____seconds and look for the sounds of laughter around me so I can enjoy the benefits.

You now have an introduction to the six components of Workin' the TEE HEE!

Do you see how they blend together in one plan? Can you identify how being cool, calm, and productive is not about an extensive list of "to-do's" but is about an intentional way of living?

I support your efforts to bring forth a cool, calm, and productive you wherever you show up each day. Keep Workin' the TEE HEE and bring forth...A Healthier You!

About The Author

Lynn Shaw, MSW

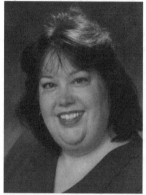

Lynn Shaw connects people to possibilities so that they can transform from tired to terrific! She strategizes with organizations to create positive energy in the workplace and increase employee satisfaction. With a rich twenty-five-year history in healthcare, mental health, business, and community service, Lynn's life applications refresh and renew from the inside out for lasting impact.

Lynn is past president and a four-year Board member of the National Speakers Association of Indiana. Other professional memberships include the Association for Applied and Therapeutic Humor, National Association of Social Workers, National Wellness Institute, and Zonta International, an executive women's service group. Lynn serves as a mental health and laughter therapy resource for news and feature stories in radio, television and magazines. Lynn holds a Master's Degree in Social Work, and she is certified in holistic stress management, Gestalt therapy and therapeutic laughter. Lynn is the director of Lifestyle Coaching at the Olson Center for Wellness in Indianapolis, Indiana. She is the author of the book, *Tee Hee Moments* and a personal growth e-course, Laughter for the Healing Heart.

Lynn Shaw, MSW, Energizing Life, Inc.
Phone: 317.691.9948
E-mail: lynn@lynnshaw.com
www.lynnshaw.com

Chapter 5

Are our kids eating themselves to DEATH?
An epidemic with only one real solution.

Dr. Dallas Humble

INTRODUCTION

In a mere twenty years—from 1980 to 2000—the prevalence of obese children (ages six to eleven) more than doubled, while obese adolescents (ages twelve to nineteen) more than tripled. These staggering statistics should shock most parents into immediate action. If left unchecked, our kids could eat themselves to death.

Consider this:

- Obese kids show higher than average blood pressure, heart rate and cardiac output—in other words, they're wearing out their hearts.
- Obese kids have higher levels of glucose intolerance and insulin—in other words, they're on track to develop diabetes.
- Obese kids develop more orthopedic problems, such as tibial torsion, bowed legs and weight stress on the knees—in other words, they're straining bones, joints and tendons.
- Obese kids show a far higher incidence of heat rash and dermatitis—in other words, they're damaging their skin, the largest organ of the body.
- Obese kids suffer from poor self-esteem, negative self-image, depression and withdrawal from peers—in other

words, they suffer emotionally, which can lead to a myriad of problems throughout their shortened lives.

The obesity epidemic can no longer be denied, ignored or blamed on someone else. My question to you is simple: What are YOU going to do about it?

As the founder of **YoungSlim Kids**™ and **The YoungSlim Lifestyle**™ (www.youngslim.com) *and* more importantly, the parent of three, I challenge you to carefully read the information contained in this chapter. I purposely prepared it in a straightforward, easy-to-digest format that will educate you and can be shared with your children. Read it as if your life depends on it—because it does.

A GUARANTEED TICKET TO FAILURE

The overwhelming body of evidence collected through countless studies points to one undeniable reality: diets don't work. Furthermore, fads don't work and crazy exercise programs don't work. Weight-loss attained through any of these three methods almost invariably returns in greater quantities within a short time after the dieting or working out stops which further results in loss of confidence, a sense of failure and the unwillingness to try again.

Thirty percent of all students think of themselves as overweight, while forty-three percent report trying to lose weight. With numbers like these, we as parents must figure out a permanent solution, or face the harsh reality that our children will resort to their own devices. Do you know what the preferred method of weight loss is rapidly becoming?

Smoking.

That's right. Our kids turn to cigarettes (and other things) as a method of weight control. Guess what? Not only will smoking lead to a plethora of other diseases, it *doesn't even work* as a weight loss method and causes a decrease in proper nutrition and physical activity—a complete lose-lose situation.

We must face the music.

The only real solution to the obesity crisis lies in a lifestyle change—and it starts with us.

WHAT CAN WE CHANGE?

The only non-changeable cause of obesity is genetics. Children of obese parents face a greater risk than others, both biologically and behaviorally. Everything else we can modify, to include:

- Physical activity and the lack thereof.
- Sedentary behavior caused by television, video games, and computers.
- Eating habits of every kind, time of day, type of food, frequency of meals, snacks and so on.
- The environment itself—overexposure to mass advertising, junk or fast food availability, access to recreational activities.

At the risk of sounding repetitive, we need to put our focus on lifestyle and behavior modification that leads to a new, healthier style of living. Nothing else will produce lasting change.

The rest of this chapter will lay out a permanent solution that you and your loved ones can embrace.

WE NEED YOUNGSLIM KIDS

For a lifestyle change to work for kids, we need to involve them, make it fun, playful, and easy to understand. Forget about austerity and painful sacrifice. That's the main reason diets don't work. They focus on deprivation—what you cannot eat, or stringent requirements that doom their duration from the beginning.

As a health care practitioner for more than twenty years, I have reviewed, evaluated and been asked about every fad, every diet, every new and revolutionary health program that has achieved even the smallest amount of notoriety.

I have seen them all.

Caring individuals who truly want to help others have created many wonderful programs. Unfortunately, for the most part, these programs don't work.

They don't work because they are too complicated.

They don't work because they are too hard to follow.

They don't work because they address only part of the problem.

They simply don't work.

What we need is a lifestyle change that even our children can embrace starting from any age and we need to begin to move in the direction of a more vibrant life without any kind of extreme behavior.

We need to address weight-management from an integrated, wellness perspective that takes into account all of the major factors that keep us young and slim.

We need to build a program that helps each person, adult or child do a little bit better in each area so that in the aggregate, the results compound and make an enormous, overall difference.

That's exactly what we have done. *The YoungSlim Lifestyle* ™ breaks down the five critical areas that must be attended to in order to help our children regain their youthful exuberance: diet, nutrition, stress, sleep, and exercise.

If we learn a little bit more about what foods to avoid, a little bit more about what foods provide great nutrients, a little bit more about how much damage can be caused by too much stress or a lack of sleep, and a little bit more about the real benefits of exercise, we can embrace these five areas in a simple, easy-to-follow program that will shed inches and pounds from our lives.

It will happen almost overnight.

DIET—THE BIG FAT LIE

Most of us love to eat. Our kids love to eat. We love the communion of breaking bread with the people that we love. It brings us together, makes us feel good. For centuries, the dining table has brought us comfort, forged relationships and created a place for dialogue. All of that is good.

Unfortunately, somewhere along the way, we moved from *eating for life*, a nurturing and growing space to *living to eat,* a space of overindulgence, ill health and yes, getting biologically older and much heavier at a premature time.

In America, we face a crisis of obesity at all levels from the elderly to our children and everyone in between. Youth are more overweight than ever, more sedentary than at any time in history and more prone to the attacks of the mass media that paint distorted pictures about health. We have become a society that feasts on junk and it shows.

What can we do? First of all, we need to understand the big fat lie.

THE BIG FAT LIE

As a concerned parent, you pick up a wrapped product and begin to read the label (your kids don't even bother). You see that it contains eight fat grams, 300 calories and twenty grams of sugar.

Based on that information, you buy the product, believing that the eight fat grams are all that you need to worry about. That is what the manufacturers want you to believe. What you don't know is that the product contains eight fat grams only when it is sealed in its wrapper.

What happens when it goes into your body is a completely different story. Guess what? We only need so much sugar for energy. When we eat products that contain sugar, the excess sugar has nowhere to go. It will convert into FAT. Therefore, a product containing only eight fat grams in its wrapper, may convert into far more fat grams in your body.

Consider a piece of hard candy. We are deceived into believing that because it contains little or no calories in the wrapper will make it non-fattening in our body. Not so at all. The sugar in the hard candy can only go one place. It converts into fat storage in our system.

The joke's on us—literally.

To compound the problem, the number of servings tricks us. We glance at the label information, log the number of fat grams and calories, and consume the product. We forget to pay attention to the number of servings. If a product has five servings in a bag, it has five times the number of fat grams and calories listed on the label—*before* the conversion of the additional sugar. We get slammed with a double-whammy and it sticks to us like a rubber tire.

We buy into the Big Fat Lie.

Now that we understand the deception, let's get into some specifics.

The bottom line is this: we have to find alternatives to the three bandidos—the three robbers—that steal our youth and our waistline and do the most damage.

ROBBER NUMBER ONE—PROCESSED SUGAR

Processed sugar is everywhere. The obvious sources such as candy and sweets represent only the tip of the iceberg. Fast food chains put sugar in the French fries, top them off with salt, and then *combine them with a toy* to addict our children. We become addicted and crave more and more. Sauces, dressings, and toppings of all types—all of these contain gobs of sugar. We already know what happens to those gobs.

Perhaps the worse offenders are soft drinks. Carbonated beverages contain ridiculous amounts of processed sugar, anywhere from twenty to as much as forty-five grams per serving. If you drink them, you know what will happen because of the Big Fat Lie. If you let your children drink them, you know what will happen. That's right. Expect the fat to accumulate.

What about diet soft drinks? The Big Fat Lie continues. The chemicals in diet drinks have been linked to degenerative diseases such as Alzheimer's. Not only that, diet drinks don't satisfy the craving for sugar. How many times have you seen a teenager order a diet drink with their banana split or mountain of chips and salsa (usually chock full of sugar as well)? Too often to remember.

Without satisfying our craving, even when we drink a diet soft drink, we reach for alternate sugar sources, trapped in an endless fat producing cycle.

If we do not manage and reduce our processed sugar intake, we can develop hyperglycemia or excess glucose in the blood stream. In addition to the weight gain, excess sugar will increase the risk of developing life-threatening conditions that range from heart disease and stroke, to blindness, nerve damage and depression.

What are your kids worth?

ROBBER NUMBER TWO—WHITE FLOUR

White flour contains no nutritional value whatsoever. Furthermore, it sits in our system like paste, congesting us and robbing us of clarity and energy. How many times have you felt that lump in your belly after a white bread sandwich? Don't mistake that for hunger satisfaction. It is no more than a blob in your stomach that your body will need to digest and expel. You gain no benefit from it. It bogs down your system, taxes your digestion and accumulates in all the wrong places.

White flour includes white bread, white pasta and white rice—all of them good for only one thing—gaining weight.

ROBBER NUMBER THREE—SALT

We need only two pounds of salt per year to function at ideal physical levels. On average, we consume ten times that much.

When we take in more salt than we need, our bodies have to compensate by retaining water to hold the salt in solution. We feel bloated and swollen *for no reason* other than reaching for the saltshaker. Too much salt leads to high blood pressure, fatigue, poor digestion, sleeplessness, nervous twitches, and a general feeling of tiredness that will plague us all day long, further lead to a sedentary state, and keep our kids indoors.

If we cut down on salt and salty snacks, we will notice a difference almost immediately.

We have so much salt in our diet anyway, that we get more than enough without ever adding any. We don't even have to try and we ingest more than enough.

Bloating has to go.

Cut back on the salt.

WASH AWAY POUNDS WITH WATER

We've shed some light on the Big Fat Lie. We've identified the three *bandidos*. What can we do to fight the cravings? We return to the source of life: WATER.

If you drink water, you think less about chips, you crave a candy bar less, and you can leave the soft drinks alone.

Our body is made up mostly of water. It cleans us out. It flushes out the junk. It dramatically reduces almost all cravings.

We need to drink one-half of our body weight in ounces of water each day. Many experts generalize this with adults and say they should drink at least six to eight eight-ounce glasses of water per day. The point is we must drink plenty of water to replenish our systems and keep our fluid retention to a minimum.

Many people fear drinking too much water because they believe it might make them swell up. In fact, the exact opposite is true. We eliminate water retention by ingesting the water that will then flush us out—a critical factor for dieting.

When it comes to weight loss, the more water we drink, the less water we carry. Therefore, we need to drink a lot of water—consistently—carry a bottle everywhere, draw a smiley face on it, whatever it takes. Our kids need water.

WE NEED GOOD FUEL

How important is proper nutrition to your body?

How important is gasoline to your car?

How important is electricity to your house?

If you feed your children foods with low levels of necessary nutrients, they will have to work much harder to extract what they need—on a daily basis.

In order to help our kids stay slim, we need to give them the proper amounts of foods both easy to digest and full of good nutrients. What do we need to know and do? Simple is best. The key is to gravitate as much as we can toward whole foods and away from processed foods.

Our nutritional needs come mostly from raw foods. That's why the American Cancer Society's health poster shows mountains of fruits and vegetables. Unfortunately, most of us don't want to eat raw foods—especially not our kids. They'd rather have fat or sugar—or both. We all know that fat tastes good in many forms. The problem is that the short-term taste benefit converts into long-term excess weight that we then carry around.

Think about it. Imagine that you decide to put five-pound weights in each of the front and back pockets of your trousers and lug them everywhere. Think of how much extra work you would have to do just to get around. Think about how much extra strain you put on your joints and muscles. As a result of this extra work, you feel fatigue and decide to boost your system with a cheap sugar product, like a candy bar. You get a sugar rush, followed thereafter by a sugar crash. Worse than the crash are the long-term effects. The sugar has nowhere to go. It will convert into more fat. You then add more weights to your pockets and carry them continuously. The stress and strain become even greater. Our desire to exercise diminishes. The vicious cycle perpetuates itself. This is precisely how our kids become obese, with no way out.

NATURE'S CANDY

We need fiber for cleansing. What is the best source? Vegetables. They contain fiber and hydrate us. Where else can we find it? Fruit, and they also hydrate our body naturally. We should be eating between five and thirteen servings of uncooked fruits and vegetables per day. That's a challenge. *Most of us won't do it.*

BUILDING MUSCLES

What about protein? You need no more than a serving that fits in the palm of your hand, once or twice each day. Chicken or fish digest more easily than red meat and fish contain essential fatty acids that lower the risk of heart disease.

Think about the consequences of excess. Whatever you don't need must be processed and expelled. That takes tremendous energy. Whatever is not expelled must be stored somewhere and in some form. What form will the storage take? Fat, fat, and more fat, the only form of storage that our body knows.

MEAL TIME IS SLIM TIME

We also need to pay attention to when we eat. If we need around 2000 calories for ideal functioning according to leading nutritionists, then obviously, when we consume them can have an enormous impact on weight loss.

If we help our kids consume eighty percent of their calories at breakfast and lunch and only twenty percent after 4 P.M., this will greatly help with weight loss.

On the other hand, if we eat very little early in the day and wait until late to consume eighty percent of our calories, then we have no time left to burn those calories. This leads to weight gain. The same 2000 calories, depending on when we ingest them, can contribute to either weight loss or weight gain according to our choices of meal times.

What else can we do to fight the tendency to over-eat late? Eat more slowly. Our body has an appetite indicator, which like a thermostat, controls our appetite. It tells us when we are hungry and continues to function for about twenty minutes after we eat our first bite. If we develop the habit of eating slowly, after twenty minutes, we will no longer feel hungry and will eat for pleasure, not to satisfy a craving.

We must find a way to moderate our food intake or we will wear out our equipment prematurely.

WHOLE FOODS VERSUS SYNTHETIC

Certain types of nutrition will aid us in fighting weight-loss, both for ourselves and for our children.

If we can't eat five to thirteen servings of raw fruits and vegetables, we still need to find a way to get the Recommended Daily Allowance (RDA) of basic vitamins and minerals. How? We can go synthetic. Whole foods mean foods made by nature. Synthetic means foods made by man. Nothing will replace whole foods though certain synthetics can help. We need a supplement to replace the lack of fruits and vegetables or to augment our intake for optimum performance. We can ingest vitamins, minerals and anti-oxidants in supplement form to help us get what we need.

If we teach our kids while young, they'll carry the habit forever.

One last recommendation—drink a glass of water before you eat. It will help curb your appetite and hydrate you at the same time.

YOUR SECRET WEAPON—THE FREE DAY

It's almost impossible to eat right every day. We get tired of the grind and we want to indulge ourselves. Go ahead. Do it. Bring the kids along for their due reward. It's okay to cheat—*but only one day per week.* We call it "Free Day." Pick one day and eat whatever you want. Indulge yourself. Have some fun. Munch it up! As human beings, we need to be rewarded for our efforts. That's what Free Day is all about. You take excellent care of your body and family for six days, then get one day to feast away on favorite foods. This simple method will truly work. Pick your day and celebrate your progress.

EASY MONEY

A popular myth often suggests that eating healthy costs too much. Not true at all. In fact, a healthy diet will almost without exception lower your monetary expenditures.

- First, by eating less, you spend less.
- Second, raw foods, for the most part, cost less than packaged foods.
- Third, healthy eating will promote better health.

You will have less physical challenges, less visits to doctors and pediatricians, lower medical bills, not to mention the lost time taken up by unnecessary healthcare issues.

SLEEP—CAN IT HELP YOU MELT?

How many times have you found yourself dragging in the middle of the day? How often do you wish you had more energy? Do you suffer from mid-afternoon malaise, a sudden desire to take a nap? What about your kids? How many times have they become grumpy or grouchy for no reason other than sheer exhaustion?

Most of us go through bouts with tiredness, sometimes for extended periods. We can't seem to get enough rest. We use willpower to somehow "make it through." Although most of us can survive a sleepy day, we should never confuse survival with functioning well, burning fat or living dynamically. The difference is immense.

Think about it. Our bodies need six to eight hours of sleep per night to function at optimal levels.

Let's run through the potential challenges:

STILL OUR BEATING HEARTS

Our heart beats at a steady rate as we rest. It, too, during sleep time has a chance to rejuvenate. During our active day, it beats at varying rates, depending on what activities we engage in, what emotions we have to deal with and so on.

We have much less stress while we sleep. If we deprive our heart of rest, it weakens and needs to pump much harder to move our blood around.

What's the result? We suffer from high blood pressure and the consequences that come with it including lethargy, little or no activity and consequent weight gain.

If we continue to forego sleep, over time the muscle becomes significantly weakened. We then need even more sleep to gain the same benefit that we used to receive with a healthy body. The downward spiral feeds itself.

Almost all of us have "gone until we dropped" at one time or another. What does that mean? It means that we have pushed ourselves until our bodies refused to go any further, refused to give us any more energy, and shut down from sheer exhaustion or total depletion of fuel. Talk about wear and tear. The effects compound within themselves. The heart has to work harder to accomplish the same result. The digestive system has to work harder to extract the same amount of nutrients. The immune system struggles to shield us from illness and more often than not, fails in the quest.

Every aspect of our being needs rest. We must sleep consistently to perform at any kind of respectable level. If we neglect sleep, we will pay.

EXPECT THE UGLINESS

Circles beneath the eyes, slouched posture, long face, flat hair, and pale countenance—you name it. If you don't rest, everything gets tired. Your eyelids won't even want to keep your eyes open.

That doesn't look pretty. The muscles that hold you up sag; the muscles in your face weaken. You lose the desire to exercise. You cease to care about what you eat, running from stimulant to stimulant to stay awake and from fat products to sugar to make yourself feel better "since you feel so wasted."

Pay attention to that word: "wasted." Is that any way to describe the way you want to feel? Is that the way you want to look? Will you let that happen to your kids?

AT THE END OF THE DAY

Consider potential bad habits. Our children stay up watching TV, become engrossed in a movie, sporting event or show that gears up their system. They then have difficulty calming back down, reach for food or a drink. Surfing the Internet can have the same effect. Video games jack them up and create the same problems.

As you can see, the principles are beginning to integrate into each other. Diet plays into nutrition. Proper nutrition gives us energy and protects us from illness. Sleep allows the body to recover and become strong each successive day. It all works together.

We need to begin the process of fighting weight gain in an integrated approach.

- We avoid harmful dietary foods.
- We seek out foods that truly feed us.
- And at the end of the day, we need to sleep.

BYE-BYE BELLY

Exercise helps all of us feel youthful and full of vitality. Most of us have gone through various exercise programs at different periods in our lives—dating all the way back to our early school days.

Surprisingly, few of us truly understand how exercise works. If we did, we would never stop and we would make sure our children didn't either.

Without wanting to sound over-simplistic, there are two critical types of exercise: cardiovascular and resistance training.

CARDIOVASCULAR EXERCISE—HEART LOVE

If asked what cardiovascular exercise means, most of us would answer simply "it's good for the heart." While correct in principle, this response in no way explains how or why cardiovascular exercise helps our heart.

Very few of us could actually explain the mechanics. If more of us knew the how and why, we would never neglect this critical component to maintaining our youth and our waistline.

Here is how it works: we begin some form of training—jogging, walking, doing aerobics or cycling and through that exercise we increase the rate at which our heart beats per minute. This process exercises the heart muscle. We must sustain the increased heart rate in order to gain the maximum benefit. Through this exercise the heart muscle gets stronger.

The true benefit doesn't happen until later, after the exercise has been completed. With a stronger muscle, the heart needs to beat fewer times per minute to flow the same amount of blood through our systems.

Through cardiovascular exercise we can build the heart muscle to a point where each beat produces the same blood flow that used to require a beat and a half, or even two beats.

A strong heart muscle translates to a longer, healthier, and more active life which means a greater level of physical activity that in turn burns more calories and keeps the weight off.

To stay young and slim, we need a healthy heart.

LIFT WEIGHTS, LOSE WEIGHT

Weight training, isometrics with rubber bands, push-ups or any exercise that puts resistance against the muscles, is called resistance training. In so doing, we actually tear down the muscle one fiber at a time. A substance called lactic acid builds inside the muscle. Lactic acid is released to provide fuel when our body runs out of glucose. The muscle then rebuilds itself stronger than before, more able to hold and flow blood—and burn more calories.

As we tone the muscles and increase the ability of the blood to be stored there, this in turn increases the size or hardness of the muscle. More muscles lead to less fat.

Active kids who climb trees, swim, wrestle and so on, are naturally doing resistance training—and they need to.

THE MAGIC TRIO

For adults, three sessions each week of cardio and resistance training will generate tremendous results. Our kids can naturally do more.

Why are both of these forms of exercise more crucial today than ever? Our society has changed. Children used to spend much more time outdoors. Now they sit on computers. Our children used to come home from school and beg to go outside. Now they rush to video games or the Internet.

Recess used to include monkey bars and jungle gyms. Now, the computer lab is packed. This physical inactivity further contributes to the epidemic of childhood obesity.

As adults our fast-paced society keeps us from spending time outdoors. We have become a fast food society, a society that chooses to "blow through a drive through" rather than take the time to eat well.

French fries are the most consumed vegetable in the country. Societal chaos leads to stress, poor eating habits lead to fatigue, lack of exercise leads to weight gain. We don't prioritize our health until it fails, at which point it may be too late. We can't afford to wait. We need an exercise program for the life-style we lead now. That program combines cardiovascular and resistance training. It only takes three sessions per week!

STRESS WEIGHT

Our children deal with one primary source of stress—problems in relationships. We deal with many more—finances, health and so on. Almost all of us can relate to hard times. Most of us have had relationships fail, from kindergarten on. We all know the sleepless nights, the worry, and the dark tunnel that seems to have no light. We have all felt stress.

The problem is, we can't see it. We can't grab hold of it and quantify it. However, we can measure its effects. We can't see the wind, but we can see the effects when it blows. Stress is the same way and when it comes to stress, the effects are not pretty.

Here's the brutal truth: **Stress can make you fat!** When stress increases, all kinds of damage takes place.

INCREASED BLOOD PRESSURE

How many of us have a family member who has had a heart attack? Most of us have, especially since heart disease is one of the major causes of death today. Increased blood pressure will wear our heart out. The extra load placed on the heart muscle hurts us both in the short term and long term. Short term, we can become short of breath, exhausted without any obvious reason, generally weak and without any desire to exercise. Long term, we risk a heart attack or stroke, almost like playing Russian roulette with our health.

WEAKENED IMMUNE SYSTEM

Our immune system governs our ability to fight off disease. Most of us know that. What we don't know is that a weakened immune system can lead to a lack of nutrient absorption. If we can't get the nutrients, our ability to recover also decreases, our strength diminishes, and our body has to work harder to get the same results that under normal conditions require much less effort.

This cycle will wear us out. At first, the immune system loses its Pacman-like ability to eat diseased cells. This leads to increased susceptibility to sickness. As soon as we get sick, a diminished immune system affects our ability to process the nutrients we need. End result? The body shuts down, exhausted.

While this may be exactly what the body needs, the damage of repeating the cycle becomes obvious. Stress makes us sick. Sickness wears us out, keeps us in bed, and out of the game.

UNNECESSARY UGLINESS

Stress affects our outward appearance in an enormous way. We get stress lines, wrinkles, bags and circles around our eyes. We see the effects mostly on the face, where it is hard to hide the effects. We compound the problem because under stress most of us—and our kids—will overeat and overindulge. We tend to stop exercising. Notice how insidious the process becomes, adding layer upon layer of strain, and fat, on our body. First we stress out. Then we stop gaining nutrients because of poor nutritional habits. We stop exercising and pack on the pounds. And then we wonder why our clothes don't fit!

DAMAGED INTERNAL ORGANS

We already talked about the heart. Unfortunately, other organs also become severely affected by stress. How many of us have digestive challenges under stress? Our stomach hurts, we experience constipation, we get heartburn.

Net effect? The body loses vitality and resilience.

Everyone knows people who look much younger than their biological years. Conversely, we know even more people who look prematurely old. One of the main reasons for premature weight gain is excess stress. *We must find ways to manage it and keep it under control.*

BALANCE—The fountain of youth!

We all want to look and feel young and we want our kids to feel that way as well. We all wish that with a magic pill we could regain that youthful vitality from our teens and keep our children from ever losing it. Unfortunately, there is no such pill. Most of us have tried one diet or another. Most of us have embarked on an exercise program. Most of us have given our children advice only to have it thrown in our faces.

Let's face it. Sticking to anything is hard. Sticking to a difficult program is almost impossible. Few of us have the discipline or tenacity to grit out anything we don't absolutely have to do—especially not at a young age. That's why a simple balance can change the life of your entire family so radically.

It's not about a tough workout regimen. It's not about eating all the same things or depriving your loved ones. Balance consists of accepting yourself as you are, wherever you are, no matter what you weigh, how tired you feel or how you look, and building little by little in the five key areas: diet, nutrition, stress management, sleep and exercise. We must lead by example for our children and teach them to do the same.

IN SUMMARY

Nothing set forth in this chapter is revolutionary. What makes it so unique is that it sets forth a basic program that anyone, especially our kids, can embrace at any time, no matter what their current condition, and gain both immediate and long term benefits that lead to permanent youthfulness.

Remember, it doesn't matter where you are today. All you need to do is start and do a little bit more than you are currently doing. It has been said that for the first time in history the possibility exists that our next generation could live a shorter life span than we have if we don't do something to combat the obesity crisis. I am urging all of you who have taken the time to read this chapter to become part of the revolution against obesity in our children. It is a mission that we all should take part in.

When you change your lifestyle as we indicate doing in the YoungSlim™ program you will feel a difference within a week and your life will change dramatically within ninety days. Do it for yourself, your children, and those you love. Not only will your life change physiologically but you will enjoy the emotional benefits of seeing those you love make positive changes in their lives as well.

About The Author

Dr. Dallas Humble

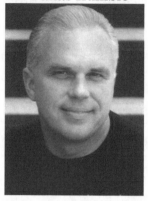

Dr. Humble earned his Doctor of Chiropractic (D.C.) degree from Palmer University in Davenport, Iowa in 1982. He has owned and operated multiple health care offices in various states overseeing doctors and their staff in the treatment and management of their patients. Dr. Humble is a Diplomate of the American Board of Anti-Aging Health Professionals (ABAAHP) and served as President of his state association in 1993-1994. He presently operates several successful businesses including a national consulting firm for physicians and Louisiana Anti-Aging and Wellness Care, which delivers state of the art anti-aging care to its patients. Dr. Humble is a highly sought after speaker and writer. He has authored several books including *Make It Happen: Strategies for Obtaining Peak Performance in Your Life* and is the co-author of the book *The Young Slim Lifestyle*. This book and lifestyle program teaches you how to reverse your age, regain your sexuality, lose all the weight you want and feel young again! Dr. Humble strongly advocates proper nutrition and wellness. He has spoken to thousands of his colleagues and individuals on subjects ranging from alternative health care to inspiration and motivation.

Dr. Dallas Humble
Phone: 318.397.9680
Fax: 318.397.9627
Email: info@dallashumble.com
www.lawc.biz

Chapter 6

It's a Matter of Choice

L.E. "Lee" McLemore, Ph.D.

As a contributor of this book I wanted to give some thought as to what would make a person "A Healthier You." There are certainly several angles from which to approach this topic: medical, diet, exercise, and even the old positive mental attitude. These are all very valid approaches; however, I wanted to offer something that might be a little off of the beaten path—perhaps some suggestions that may allow you to take your thoughts to a deeper level of who you are and where you are going.

When I look at people who are "healthier" (which by the way is a subjective term), I tend to notice this *aliveness* about them, a glow if you will. They tend to move in ways that radiate confidence and purpose. Even those who have been diagnosed with a particular disease seem to take it with a grain of salt and simply move into a space of self-healing. It is as though they are very aware of why they are on this planet and are very committed to their mission and vision. There is an extra lilt in their step, an extra sparkle in their eye, and a vibrancy that attracts others who say, "I want what they have!"

On the other hand, there are those who appear to be simply going through the motions of life. They get up every morning, go to work, come home, have diner, and watch television, then off to bed, only to do all over again, day in and day out. On the weekends they do the "Honey Do" list or work around the house.

Sunday, it's off to church, and then off to Sunday dinner, and Monday morning they start the routine all over again. This is repeated month after month, and year after year and they look up one day and realize their life is half over. They wonder what have they accomplished? How have they savored life? What have they learned? What have they loved—were passionate about? To me, this is an *unhealthy life*.

Several months ago, before I started this project, I began working on a new book. It is intended to expand on my theories and beliefs about this "alive state of being" I've been talking about. The working title is *Are you Living your Life or is your Life Living You?* I think the subject matter is very appropriate for this book, so I decided to highlight it for you here.

"Lifitis"

I have discovered a new disease, which is taking America by storm. It's called "Lifitis" (l Ī f• Ĩt es) and is defined as the "Inflammation of Life."

Etiology: Noted when one's life becomes consumed with external and internal pressures that the person begins to live an automatic life. During such time choices, options, and opportunities appear to have diminished or are completely eliminated from conscious awareness. Notable loss of passion with an increased attention spent on past and future events, thoughts, and experiences. May have a tendency to lean toward the mundane and the average vs. the challenging and invigorating. One's life becomes so inflamed with the motion of life that your life is actually living you, instead of you living your life.

Age Range: 18 – pre-Moses

Onset: Early onset noted post secondary education around or at the time of role change (i.e., going from student to employee, from young unmarried adult to married adult with responsibilities)

Late Stages: Bitterness, Regret, Blame, Loneliness, Heartache, and finally...Death.

Symptomology:

1. **Language Patterns:** Typical language patterns may include, but are not limited to: "I have to—," "I've got to—," "I should—," "He makes me feel—," "I can't believe what they did to me—," "I never—," "They always—."

2. **Feelings:** Feelings may range from overwhelmed, to complacency, to boredom, to being stuck in life, to dread, to being detached, to going through the motions.

3. **Thought Processes (may present with one or more)**
   a. *Through Time vs. In Time*: This is a filter that many of us have. When someone is in "Through Time" they are disengaged and are viewing life from the sidelines. These are the individuals who will often say, "Did we just discuss—" "What did we do this morning?" "I'm sorry, what did you just say?" When someone is "In Time," they are present and actively participating on all levels.
   b. *Past, Future vs. Present*: Those who are stuck in "Past" and "Future" tend to focus on events that happened in the past and might happen in the future. They will say things like: "At my last job—" "The way we used to do this—" "One day I will—" "Once I get X then I'll feel Y." Those who focus on the here and now are Present: In Time.
   c. *Muddled Thinking*: This is self-explanatory. Those who experience muddled thinking simple find themselves focusing on a task, unable to get their thoughts organized. They tend spend a lot of time thinking and contemplating and staring off into space.
   d. *Unclear thoughts*: The kissing cousin to Muddled Thinking. Unclear thoughts, is simply when you have difficulty deciding how you think or feel about a given situation, thought or idea.

4. **Behaviors (may present with one or more)**
   a. *Stressed:* May be noted by short temper, snappy responses, unusually quietness, or an overall shutdown.
   b. *Poor time management*: Difficulty getting tasks completed, unable to focus on tasks, never having enough time to complete tasks, a tendency to push deadlines back due to lack of time.
   c. *Living life out of balance*: Notable imbalance of Work, Play, Rest, and Sleep.

> d.   *Unable to set or execute outcomes,* unaware of or
>   inability to set goals and find direction, a ten-
>   dency to get off track when in pursuit of a goal.

Those who meet sixty percent or higher of the above criteria
are to be considered suffering for Lifitis. Simply stated: They are
not living their life, but instead, their life is living them.

All right, I'm sure you've figured it out by now that I'm having
a little fun with you, however, I do believe that we have a very
serious problem today. Many in our society meet some of the criteria I've laid out and their life is truly living them. What about
you—is your life living you or are you living your life?

Sleepwalking

Criminals on death row are called a "dead man walking" as
they walk down the hallway going toward the execution chamber.
Although they are living, breathing, walking down the hall, and
they have the ability to enjoy conscious thought, they are still
considered "DEAD."

Well, I'm not as harsh with my label of people; however, I believe that the majority of our society is "sleepwalking." They are
alive, breathing, talking, walking, eating, interacting, moving
through life's motions, etc., however, they are still asleep and are
passively living life.

Now we have two ends of the spectrum here. You have one
side: The Zombies. Yes, that's right, The Zombies. They are the
ones you see walking around the supermarket and in the mall
with no expression. They appear to be going through life somewhat detached. Now, the good thing about zombies is that they
roll with the punches. They have a very high stress tolerance and
nothing seems to bother them. They are neither moody nor elated.
They take things with a grain of salt and typically can't be
swayed one way or another. Not because they are grounded in
who they are, and what they know, but because they don't stand
for anything. Therefore you can persuade them to see your point
of view very easily. The challenge is they can be easily persuaded
to someone else's point of view as well.

The other end of the spectrum is the "Super Engaged." These
people are harder to spot because they appear to have it all together. You will look at them and say. "Wow, what a terrific mom!
She is involved in all of the kids' activities," or, "What a terrific
employee! He is here every morning at 8:30 at this desk and

working." Yes, the people in both of these examples have great attributes but are they truly awake or are they *Sleepwalkers?*

The answer lies within the consciousness of their involvement of their activities. If they are living their lives by *should do's, need to's,* and *got to's,* then they are Sleepwalking; however, if they have made a conscious choice to engage in their kids activities, not because "it's the thing to do," or, "my child's friends are all signing up for baseball, then I guess I need to sign up my child as well." The conscious choice is when your child comes up to you and says, "I want to play ball," and you can quickly identify the needs, values, and purpose the sport will play in your child's life as well as the family unit.

Sleepwalkers are also those who are going day after day, week after week, and month after month without considering or setting their goals. With the clients whom I see, one of the first issues we must come to an agreement about is what are we working on. I don't see clients just to see them or allow clients to keep booking appointments just because they enjoy the session. What are we working on, and what is it that we want to accomplish?

I would hope that you would not get in your car and take a vacation without knowing where you are going. You may not have a road map (which we can talk about in another book) but you should have some idea of where you want to go. So tell me why would you get into the biggest vehicle of all—your body—and take a journey down the longest road—your life—without knowing where you are going?

In the spirit of Jeff Foxworthy during his "You must be a redneck when—" routine, let me see if you can identify with these:

You must be Sleepwalker—

- When you wake up every day without goals and directions.
- When you go down the journey of life and don't know where you're going.
- When you can't identify the pleasure, joy and passion from your day.
- You look back over the last five years and can't figure out where you've spent your time.
- When you wake up one day and find out you life is over because you forgot to start.

It's time to wake up and make your dreams your reality.

Waking Up

What I mean by "waking up" is when you have come to the point in your life when you begin to realize that there must be more. You begin to question the WHY in everything you do: Why do I have this job? Why do I live here? Why do I wear the blue suit on Tuesdays? Why do I always wake, go to the bathroom, and brush my teeth, then shower every morning? Why don't I wake up, shower, and then brush my teeth? Why? Why? Why? It's that questioning of belief systems, patterns, habits, and who we are that helps us begin to wake up.

It started for me one Sunday morning, while living on the top floor of an Atlanta high rise. I woke up from a usual night "on the town" and realized that there must be something more. I had the car, the apartment and the job, but what did I have to show for it? Nothing. I'm not talking about physical acquisitions—I'm talking about that sense of being. I remember feeling the emptiness and peace at the same time. The emptiness was from the realization that although I had everything I thought I wanted, I had nothing, and the peace was from knowing that I was going to be okay and it was time for the next chapter of my life.

You may experience this awakening through a multitude of experiences, ranging from the subtle nudging of your inner feelings to experiencing a catastrophic event. The experience can be as gentle as you desire or as cathartic as you need. The bottom line is: one day, life as you know it has or will change. Remember, you may go through several stages of the awakening throughout your life.

What are we awakening to? Well, our religious organizations would say that we are awakening to Christ or the Christ energy or perhaps being aware that it is time to "make Jesus Christ you personal Lord and Savior." The metaphysical community will contend that you are waking up to the "light"—to the energy of universal life force—the chi, if you will. Others may say you are waking up to your inner knowing, your collective consciousness, or perhaps you super- consciousness. And to all of that I say, *"Yes!"* You see, whatever you call your higher self, your God essence, or you higher power is fine, because it is *your* path and *your* awakening. Whether you pray to Jesus, Buddha, Allah, Mother Mary, or any of the other deities I left out, it is perfectly all right.

It is my belief that these are all facets of the same. This supreme energy has many faces and many aspects, so the entire world may have that connection—that familiarity. You see, I don't feel there is one path or road map to "the light" or to "God." If that were true, we would all be the same with all of the same issues and challenges. We are created with various backgrounds, various lessons to learn in life and various opportunities to explore. That's what makes life so wonderful—to know that no matter how different we are, we are all looking for and fighting for the same thing.

I mean, isn't that why wars are fought? Both opponents, at some level, want the same thing: the same piece of land, or the same pot of gold, or the same religious freedom, etc. The only difference is that we are on different paths and road maps to get it! Wow! What would happen if we realized that we all wanted the same thing, but instead of making the other person right or wrong (because "You don't want to do it my way") we would help others achieve their goals and journeys and by doing that, we may achieve our own. Is that not a healthier perspective?

"Through the serving of others may my dreams truly come true." You see, "no man is an island." You've heard these clichés before. The fact remains that we are all connected—we are all part of the same. If you want to get scientific about it, everything on the inside is relatively the same. The difference is the color of our skin and the six inches between our ears.

Waking up is gaining the knowing that there is something bigger than you are; that there is something more—something beyond us—yet inside us at the same time. Waking up is the realization that the mission and the journey of life goes beyond our imagination; to find out what our role is within it; that is our challenge.

Rediscovering Self

The first step in discovering self, or re-discovering self (for those who went back to sleep) is of course answering the question, "Who are you?" If you have read any of my other writings or attended any of my lectures or courses, you will find this section familiar. This is one of the most critical steps to discovering self and to begin living with passion and purpose.

In this culture we have taken on the identity of our beliefs, our capabilities, our behaviors, and our environment to be the true essences of "who we are." We have become so accustomed to labeling things and people that it has become second nature. By placing labels on things and people, we are able to put them in a box and when we put things in a box, then we will know how to relate to them, what to expect from them, and most notably, how to separate and categorize them.

He is a doctor so he must be the authority in his field of medicine. He will have all the answers and now I no longer have to take responsibility for my health, I can rely on the doctor. Here we have mistaken a man's capabilities for his identity.

She is a CEO so she is the person in charge of this company, responsible for its growth and therefore is directly responsible for the amount of my paycheck. Oh, and by the way, a *woman* as a CEO? Well, there is another set of prejudged thought processes that go with that such as: She's probably not a good mother because she spends her time at work; she is a man-eater, cold, and a some other descriptors that I dare not include. Here again we have mistaken her environmental role as her identity and then added our own preconceived meaning of what type of person she may or may not be; yet we know nothing about *her*.

With these boxes into which we place people come certain perceived roles and responsibilities that goes with that box. But where did we come up with those roles and responsibilities? Our cultural influences? Perhaps. Our parents or religious affiliation? Perhaps. Or it could be that we just decided in our own mind this is the way we like it and we believe this is the way it should be. All points of view are right and there is no wrong perspective *until* we begin to impose our beliefs on to others.

To discover "who you are," you need to begin to remove your "self" from your job. You are not your job. You need to remove your self from your behaviors. You need to challenge your beliefs and see which are serving you and which are limiting you.

I'm always reminded of the story (whether true or made up) of the little girl who, at Sunday dinner, asked her mother why she cut off the ends of the roast before putting it in the oven.

The mother replied, "I don't know, that's the way my mother did it. Go in and ask your grandmother who is the living room."

The little girl went and asked the grandmother, "Why do we cut of the ends of the roast before we put it in the oven?"

The grandmother replied, "I don't know, that's the way my mother did it. Let's give Granny a call and ask her."

So they called Granny who was about ninety-eight years old and asked "Why do we cut of the ends of the roast before putting it in the oven?

Granny replied, "I don't know why *you* do it, but I did it because it wouldn't fit in my roasting pan."

That little bit of humor was to make a point. What we do and who we are is because of unconscious choices we make based on our lineage, culture, and religious upbringing. There is no judgment of right or wrong, it just is.

Now the question is, "Who are *you*?" Do your beliefs, behaviors, and feelings serve you or not? If not, then you need to make some choices and changes.

By understanding who we are and by removing the boxes from around our identity will help us gain clarity on our reality. Part of "Waking Up" is realizing that that the world we live in is not necessarily our reality—it is an illusion of our mind based on our own maps and filters.

The second step in rediscovering yourself is answering the questions, "Why are you here?" Or better yet, "What is your purpose?" Ah! Yes, the age-old question, but one that will set you on your path of a healthier and more meaningful existence. I believe that you can't answer the second question until you answer the first. And I also believe that these questions are to be answered in layers. Who I was ten years ago and who I am today has evolved. No, I didn't say changed, but evolved and who you were and whom you will be will also evolve.

Are you here to teach, to be a healer, to motivate, to orchestrate, to lead, to serve, or even to follow? You see, there is no right or wrong, it *your* purpose. The best way to find out *your* purpose, or at least to get started on that path, is to spend some time with yourself and get in touch with what excites you. What makes you get up in the morning? What is the first thing you think of when you get up? What is the last thing you think of when you go to bed at night? The answers to these questions are what I call "clues." The answers you give will show you what your passion is.

Now the next step is, how can I take this "passion" and serve humankind? That's your purpose.

Understanding oneself is the key to living a healthier and more prophetic life. If you know who you are, what you stand for, then you can easily move into what your purpose is. Now that you have rediscovered yourself, you are ready to begin your conscious living.

Conscious Living

Okay, I'm sure you're thinking, "Aren't we all living consciously?" Well no. You see, there are those who have been sleepwalking, those who have begun to wake up and realize there is something more, and then there are those who realize there is more but are being driven by their unconscious patterns or habits. Well, now it is time to begin to learn how put things into motion—how to question our unconscious programs and make some conscious choices.

We are the accumulation of all the experiences we have had since birth. Actually, there are studies that suggest that we are even receptive to communication while in utero. Parents are even encouraged to talk to their unborn child during pregnancy. Playing soothing music will calm a child prior to its birth. Some people actually feel that they are the product of their grandparent and grandparents before them. It might even be safe to say that recent studies with energetic DNA show we are a product of our entire lineage from the beginning of time. Well, regardless of which "jumping off" point you choose to believe for your reality, you cannot deny that you have some personality traits, behaviors, and/or habits that are identical to your ancestors.

I believe one of the most common examples is that of new parents who say, "I'm not going to make the same mistakes my parents did." Or better yet, siblings who state, "I can't believe you are raising your child that way," only to find out after they have *their* first child, some of the same patterns of behaviors emerge.

Everyone has good intentions and they set out to do the best possible job (and they do) yet they tend to experience behaviors from time to time that are reminiscent of the way their parents behaved. Why? Well, because, they have their parents' DNA. They have the experience of a similar situation in their being, and on the time line. When they encounter this similar experience, then the automatic reactions take over.

I like to talk about this as a "program of patterns." You see, within our being we have millions of these programs that I like to call "probabilities" or "potentialities." They are lying dormant until they are triggered. Like a fifty disk compact disk (CD) changer--there are fifty potential CDs you could play, however, you will hear nothing until you select the CD you want. Well, within our experience, there is an outside stimulus we will see, hear, or feel that will trigger our program. The challenge is that most of the CDs—programs—are unconscious. Actually, many of the triggers are outside of our awareness as well.

Our conscious mind processes more than seven bits of information plus or minus two in any given second. However, our subconscious mind processes more than two millions bits of information at any given second. Let me explain. If you were in an air-conditioned building and you went outside in 100-degree weather, you would not consciously think, "Okay, it is now hot, so I need to activate my sweat glands. I need to reach up and wipe the preparation off of my forehead. I need to grab the front of my shirt and fan it to get some cool air circulating under my shirt." No, these are automatic responses to the stimulus of heat.

Take this same theory and map it over to your day-to-day life. The tone of someone's voice could trigger a negative response from you and yet you don't know why. Have you ever said, "I just don't get a good feeling from them. Hmm, I wonder why?" Your husband comes home from work and says something or does something that triggers a story or program having to do with you and your father; you then lash out at your husband and he stands there saying, "What did I do?" These are programs that need to be removed.

I have several clients who will come in and give examples of little things they do and/or habits that they just want to get rid of. Unbeknown to them, it was these same behaviors and/or habits that their mother, grandmother, or aunt had. Although knowing where these behaviors/habits came from is not always necessary, but it does provide a story that can appease the conscious, analytical part of our being.

We go through life living each day with hundreds of these unconscious programs in our daily experience. Why? Because it is part of our genetic makeup. I'm not saying whether it is right or wrong as much as I am suggesting that this is what I call "unconscious living." Now that you are beginning to wake up to the idea that there is something greater than all of us, it's time to question these unconscious patterns or programs and see which ones are worth keeping and which ones are not serving you.

I'd like to add another caveat here—judgment. We tend to quickly move into a space where we have to place an interpretation or meaning of our exercise, especially if you are "waking up." It is all about taking stock and analyzing where you are; great, but let's do it without judgment.

The judgment I'm talking about is the right vs. wrong. Our society is so quick to assess the "wrong" in things. It is so much easier to look at what went wrong or what is wrong about something than to identify what is right. Yet the exact same experience has both, "right" and "wrong." It is at this point where you must decided what value will you get from focusing on the right vs. the wrong. I know you may say, "Well, seeing the wrong will make me a better person," and I say to that, "Possibly, and can't seeing the good in something make you a better person as well?"

You see, focusing on the wrong or the negative side creates a lower or negative vibration, and with that tends to produce shame, guilt, disappointment, you know, all of the great gifts of emotions that keep on giving. My question is, "How does focusing on the negative serve you? What benefit do you get from being in the negative space?" You can look at the same experience and see the "lesson" of the experience, and by the mere fact that you learned something, make it a positive experience.

I know this is a lot to swallow in this short chapter, and if you subscribe to this theory then you would never have another negative experience again. That may be a bit much, so take it as slow as you need. Just for now though, let's look at our behavior or patterns without judgment. They are just patterns or behavior. All we have to do is ask, "Is this behavior or pattern serving me?"

There is another piece to conscious living I would like to introduce. That is "living in the moment." We may have all heard this before and this is nothing new here, except to say, when you are totally committed to living in the moment you are fully present in your consciousness. You will have a heightened sense of awareness and it is in this space that your unconscious programs cannot be triggered.

Most of us live our life in the past or in the future. Those who are in the past will constantly be talking about what happened yesterday, what experience they had, who did what to whom, etc. Those who are in the future, are the daydreamers, the "what if'ers." They will also be the ones worrying about the bills, or wondering if everything will be okay, or when the other shoe will drop.

I won't go into a lot of stories about this angle, but I will say that if you are stuck in the past or in the future, you're missing the present. There is a great anonymous quote I enjoy and is so appropriate for this section:

"The past is a history, the future is a mystery, all we have is now, is a gift, that's why it's call the *present*."—Anonymous.

Once you begin to ask questions and evaluate your patterns, you are now in the present and consciously living. You have gained clarity of who you are, what your purpose is, and now you are taking responsibilities for all of your patterns. Perhaps now is time to learn how to create choices in your life.

"Conscious living is when you are fully present and aware of your everyday decisions, actions, and existence. Conscious living is creating choices and opportunities in life."

Creating Choices

If there is one thing I hope you understand from my rambling in this chapter, it would be, "The Power of Choice." *Everything is a choice.* Once you move into conscious living, you are able to realize that more and more decisions are by choice. When you first begin, you may find it difficult to come up with a particular choice, and that is okay, as long you acknowledge that it *is* a choice. Even having no other options is a choice, because you simply may not do or say or be. The choosing whether to do, say, or be, is in fact, a choice.

One of the most common areas I am able to catch my clients limiting their choices is within their language patterns. One area is the "Have to's," "Got to's," and the, "Should's." Wow! Right away you can see how these statements eliminate any other possibilities. I like to challenge my clients with a simple, "What if? What if you didn't do—? What would be so bad?" Even if the consequences would not be what they wanted, at least they are able to see another choice.

Another area is where my clients describe their mood. "I'm angry," "I'm so upset," "I feel depressed." Right away you can notice that these statements leave no room for choices, right? So as a rule of thumb I have them insert the words *choose to feel* or *be* in front of every emotion: "I choose to be angry." "I choose to feel upset." "I chose to feel depressed." This one technique then gives them an immediate *choice to* not "be," or "feel," and then to choose a different emotion.

What a powerful gift to offer someone—the option and permission not to feel angry upset or depressed!

Okay, I know. How can you feel something different than anger when you are angry? Remember the part about finding the positive aspect of the same situation—the lesson to be learned? What I'm talking about here is "reframing."

The art of reframing is a gift and skill all in itself. It is the ability to look at someone or something with a different frame of reference is an amazing power tool to have in your toolbox. Think about it. Comedians make a living doing this. They have the ability to take common, ordinary news items and draw different conclusions. What about the public relations profession? PR people do this all the time. What about our own U.S. Press Secretary? The truth of the matter is that any time you have more than two people experiencing the same situation, each will have their own interpretation. Are they wrong? No, each has his or her own reality. Well guess what? *You can do the same.* Practice looking at the same experience; yet come up with two different interpretations of that experience.

Here are some examples. Regarding the Iraq War: did we destroy a country or free a country? When you lost your job today: did you get fired or did you create an opportunity to find a better job? Were your emotional eruptions a negative outburst or a passionate stance? Are people who badmouth the President anti-American or patriots, because they care so much for their country that they want things to be different?

Do you get the picture? We could go on for days. Every situation has both a positive and negative side. It is your choice to choose which side is going to be *your* reality. Once you begin to see your world though choice, then you are able to open up and create endless possibilities.

I also subscribe to the belief that we have all the information within us at all times. Everything you ever need to know, you know already. The challenge is that you aren't able to access the information. Why? Because, you are focusing on the negative. The way to access your resources is to connect with your inner self— connect with that inner knowing. Trust that you *do* make the best possible decision at each moment. This doesn't mean that in two minutes from now you can access more information and might make a better decision. But at the moment of decision, you will always make the best possible choice.

A Healthier You

In my opinion, "A Healthier You" is about discovering the true essence of who you are, what your purpose is and living each day in the present moment, savoring life with every ounce of your being. The minute you begin to get off track, loose focus, and live your life because of have to, should to, and got to, then you are no longing living your life, but you life is living you.

About The Author

L. E. "Lee" McLemore, Ph.D.

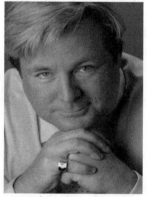

L. E. "Lee" McLemore, Ph.D., a national tele-vised trainer/speaker/author, is the president of Peak Performance Consultants, Inc, founder of the Institute of Alternative Modalities. His clients range from multi-Grammy Award winning artists, CEO's VP's to single entrepreneurs. Dr. Lee's unique talents allow him to peel back the onion to expose and resolve the key challenges that are blocking you on your journey. He assist his clients to remove, take away or dissolve what has always held them back, what has created anxiety, what has stopped them from being and doing at the level of awesome excellence that they have dreamed about or glimpsed in their reverie. "As we hold the space for change, behavior patterns shift, em-powering beliefs emerge, passionate energy flows through, and focus is on the choices that bring them to success and peace in their life in spite of nay Sayers around them. Everyone has the potential, however, some need assistance to access it". Dr. Lee believes that many can coach, but few can truly find the leverage it takes to create massive behavioral changes. His sessions are interactive and provide the arena for live prob-lem resolution. Not only do his clients learn new strategies, but also are able to experience real-life applications.

L. E. "Lee" McLemore, Ph.D.
Institute of Alternative Modalities
Phone: 404.876.5140
Fax: 404.420.2228
www.iofam.com

Chapter 7

Looking Good and Feeling Great at Any Age:
Some Things I Have Learned So Far

Gwen Herb

I. INTRODUCTION

We're All Doing It!

Each and every one of us is doing it right now. It beats the alternative. What is it? It is growing older! We can't avoid it. With the alternatives, who would want to? The longer we live, the longer most of us want to live—it is self-perpetuating—it is infectious—it feeds on itself—it can be fun and fulfilling; but it should not be approached haphazardly.

My Credentials

Why listen to what I have to say? My best friend said to me, "Why would anyone listen to you?" I was really taken aback. Self-doubt set in. I gave it a lot of thought, because my passion is health, and sharing what I have learned with others is my new purpose in life.

I am not a medical doctor. I don't even portray one on television. Obviously we need and appreciate doctors, but most doctors are oriented to treatment, not prevention. Doctors and their staffs are busy and overworked. They do not have the time available many of them wished they had to review our problems. We leave their offices disappointed in the lack of time we were given. Some doctors do not have the best bedside manners. A visit to the doctor is often intimidating just because it is a visit to the doctor. Answers we do get to our health questions are often confusing because of medical terminology, which is beyond the grasp of ordinary people to understand. In spite of this, remember that the squeaky wheel gets oiled. So get oiled—get your answer, even if it is an "I don't know." It is your body, you want it to last.

We know that doctors receive very little education on nutrition. We also know that the healthcare system in our country is in crisis. It is going to get worse if Americans don't get healthier.

My knowledge of preventive health has come from being an educated patient. While I hold no advanced degree from a university, I believe I have earned a doctorate in life experience from the hard knocks college of knowledge about health. I am a speaker for various health organizations, including the American Cancer Society, the National Osteoporosis Foundation, and the American Health Association. I've been a member of the Air Force, a flight attendant, a travel agent under the Capitol dome in Washington, a model, and a real estate broker. I've traveled the world. I now live in Boca Raton, which has given birth to the healthy meatless "Boca Burger" and is home to a growing number of health enthusiasts and organizations. I am in a perpetual state of learning by way of seminars, conventions, health magazines, Internet daily messages from various health organizations, and Internet searches. I am a long-standing member of the moms' and wives' club. Such women are on the front line in defense of family health. Women traditionally assume the role of caring for their families with love and nurturing.

Bottom line, I have sixty-six years of experience in the art of growing older. I plan to live to be 100; more importantly, I plan to enjoy those final years. My goal is to do everything possible I can to avoid a destiny of not being able to care for myself. Let me share my observations with you.

It is Never Too Early, It is Never Too Late—NOW *is* the Time!

What time is it where you are? It is never too early to take preventive steps to protect your health. It is never too late to take steps to improve a health problem. NOW *is* the time for all of us to get serious about the most precious thing we possess—our health. Time waits for no person; you need to start getting serious NOW.

Can your plan for healthy aging be described as an "ostrich syndrome," (i.e., burying your head in the sand and ignoring reality in favor of an imaginary place where everything is perfect)? Do you believe "ignorance is bliss"? That dangerous phrase is actually a misquote from an eighteenth century poet, Thomas Gray, who said "Where ignorance is bliss, 'tis folly to be wise." Ignorance is definitely not bliss where your health is concerned.

Things can appear to go well for quite a while under the "ostrich syndrome." Reality inevitably intrudes. I am reminded of the old cartoon of the man who jumps off the Empire State Building. As he passes the forty-second floor in his free fall downward, someone shouts out the window to him, "How is it going?"

The man responds, "So far, so good."

Can your health be described as "So far, so good?"

Age *is* Relative

You've probably heard the phrase, "age is relative." What does it mean? What does it mean to you? As a humorous quick fix, one way to feel younger is to hang out with older people. One way to feel thinner is to hang out with obese people.

A few years ago I returned to my hometown for my forty-fifth year class reunion. Have you recently gone to your class reunion? Isn't it amazing how everyone *else* has gotten old? The women looked pretty good, other than many had put on weight. But the men—they looked as if they did not really care. By and large, that's true. Some of them won't be around for the next reunion.

When I was in my early twenties, I thought sixty-six was really old. From my present vantage point, sixty-six seems reasonably middle-aged. Some say that "old" is anyone fifteen years older than you are. That's a notion we can all subscribe to. In any event, no matter what your current age, you don't want to become a person who says, "If I knew I was going to live so long, I would have taken better care of myself." You don't want to grow old *and* live to regret it. But what can we do? We are a society that expects instant results—instant gratification—a magic pill to cure all ills. Nevertheless, good health and longevity require preparation. Begin to prepare now.

The New Math of Aging

Humorists observe that a person's frame of reference to his or her own numeric age evolves over time. The only time in life when you like to get old is when you are a child. If you are not yet ten you are excited about aging. You think in terms of fractions such as "I'm four and a half" or "I'm six and a half." When you get to your teens, you jump to the next number—"I'm going to be 16." You then "turn" (as in bad milk) thirty, "push" forty, "reach" fifty, "make it" to sixty, and "hit" seventy. When you survive to your nineties, you start going backwards, such as, "I was just 92." If you turn the odometer to 100, you return to the child stage and again use fractions, such as, "I'm 100 and a half."

Is your biological age your "real age?" Dr. Michael F. Roizen has written a book titled *Real Age: Are You as Young as You Can Be?* He propounds forty-four steps that delay aging. He also asserts that you can exert some control over how your genes affect your health. While genes do play a part, they are not as important as our environment and as how we care for ourselves. The genetic part is about thirty percent; the rest is up to us. Even if there is a bad gene factor, by routine examinations and by keeping our immune systems strong, we can seek to combat it. Dr. Roizen has established a web site at http://realage.com. Visit the site to take his real age test. By supplying information about you, his test will adjust your biological age upward or downward—depending on your particular personal information as it relates to your health—to arrive at your "real age."

Not only is age "relative" between individuals, it is relative between generations. We are younger than our parents' generation, not just in the obvious chronological sense. Life expectancy keeps increasing. When I was born in 1938, the life expectancy was to age fifty-eight. Today, life expectancy for a woman is eighty-six. Life expectancy for a man is seventy-seven. The new equation has become that older is really younger. A sixty-year-old person today is like a forty-five-year-old person was some thirty years ago. Sixty has become the new middle age. Does that mean that we can expect to live until the age of 120? For most of us, it's unlikely, even though studies show our human DNA makeup could readily allow us to live to the age of 120.

Today, the 100 plus age group has become the fastest growing category. This is all wonderful if you are in good health for those golden years. Modern medicine has helped make that possible. The ultimate responsibility, however, is still with each of us, so that we can enjoy those years—ensure that they are golden, not constructed of fool's gold. Life is not measured by the number of breaths we take, but by the moments that take our breath away. Americans are the unhealthiest people on the planet. You need not be part of that demographic. Change the equation in your favor.

Be Your Own Mentor

How do you see yourself in five, ten, fifteen and twenty-five years from now? What does "health" mean to you? What does getting older mean to you? What's your greatest passion? What's the greatest challenge in your life? How do you go about clarifying your views on these questions?

Choices. Life is all about choices—the smart ones we make and the not so smart ones we make. Our schools need a mandatory course, "Life Choices 101." As young people, we don't think of the consequences of the choices we make. From the foods we eat, to the friends we make, to the lifestyles we choose to live. Not only have the choices become more important but life has also become riskier, more stressful, and more complicated than it ever has been. We can't do much to change the past. We can, however, learn from it. We can do a lot about our future—about how we want to be in five, ten, fifteen and twenty-five years from now. "Goal" research shows that setting goals, writing them down, and reviewing them periodically will give you the best chance of reaching a goal.

You will generally have to become your own mentor on your journey to old age. Becoming informed is necessary to enable you to embark in the right direction. Keeping informed is vital to prevention. The phrase, "an ounce of prevention is worth a pound of cure," is not accurate. It is a gross understatement of the value of prevention. Successful aging is a matter of mind—making intelligent health decisions, and having a proper attitude. Maya Angelou has said that if you don't like something, change it. If you cannot change it, change the way you think about it. Scott Friedman, president of the National Speakers' Association, has an appropriate poem about perception:

You can be just thirty-three and over the hill,
or eighty-five going on twenty-nine.
The young at heart don't care about years. They
know age is only a state of mind.
You are never too old to be young, so make love
and laughter part of the plan.
The best thing in life is to die young, as old
as you possibly can.

We all need to become educated patients. A vast amount of information is available on the Internet. For two examples, visit WebMD: http://aolsvc.health.webmd.aol.com/home/ or Medscape: www.medscape.com/today. Take a few minutes; search the Internet for various subject matters. You will be amazed at what you find. When we do consult a doctor, do not hesitate to get a second opinion. After all, doctors are only people and we need to be aware of the difference between trying to treat symptoms versus trying to treat the underlying cause of a given condition.

There is no magic pill. But a proper attitude can be magical.

Get Started on the Right Foot: A Prayer to Start the Day

I find I can have a positive attitude for good health and successful aging if I start each day with the following prayer (author unknown):

Dear Lord:
I'm proud to say, so far today,
I've got along all right;
I have not gossiped, whined or bragged
or had a single fight.
I haven't lost my temper once,
or criticized my mate;
I have not lied, I have not cried,
or loudly cursed my fate.
So far today I've not one time
been grumpy or morose;
I've not been spiteful, cold or vain,
self-centered or verbose.
But, Lord, I'm going to need Your help,
throughout the hours ahead;
So give me strength, dear Lord, for now,
I'm getting out of bed.

II. THINGS I LEARNED FROM MY MOTHER

Many of the things you hear about good health and successful aging are repeats of things you have heard many times before. Some of these things your mother told you. We all remember, "don't make faces because your face might freeze that way," or, "don't run with open scissors," or, "wear clean underwear in case you are in an accident."

The importance of paying attention to underwear became apparent to me in 1960. I was a stewardess on a Northwest Orient flight from Seattle to New York. We were flying over Chicago in the early morning hours. Most of the passengers were sleeping. I was called into the cockpit. The captain told me that our gyrocompass had gone out. I didn't know what a gyrocompass was; it certainly didn't sound like a good thing. The captain said we would need to land at the nearest airport because of our inability to navigate. We also had to jettison fuel for the landing. I had to wake the passengers to prepare for landing. We were flying a DC-8, which had first class sleeping births. One of the passengers I had to wake was Senator Henry "Scoop" Jackson (at that time he was also the Chairman of the Democratic Party, involved in managing John F. Kennedy's successful run for the presidency). When I woke him, I was surprised to see that he was sleeping in his red "jammies." He was pleasant and courteous. I was a bit embarrassed by his bedtime attire. We were able to land without incident. When Senator Jackson de-planed, he was dressed in his suit. I said the traditional, "bye-bye," and in my mind, I heard my mother saying: "Make sure you wear clean underwear, in case you're in an accident."

More directly related to health, you probably remember your mother telling you to eat the right foods, get enough rest, exercise regularly, don't do drugs, don't smoke, and don't drink alcohol to excess. I don't know about you, but I was one of those who didn't listen. I worked at a chocolate shop after school; I ate most of the profits. My favorite exercise was shopping—when I was a stewardess at eighteen I would go almost three days without sleep. I never did drugs, but I drank alcohol whenever I could get my hands on it. My mother told me that smoking would kill me. My response was that I would rather live a shorter life and enjoy myself—eventually I had to die from something. As I matured, I found that everything my mother told me was correct. After all, most of us recall from school the words of Benjamin Franklin's, *Poor Richard's Almanac,* 1758, "Early to bed and early to rise, makes a man healthy, wealthy, and wise."

I also learned from my mother as she aged. It was time to get serious about my health, or suffer all the health problems my Mother had. She had fallen and broken her hip at age fifty-nine, and again at seventy. She had two hip replacements, she had a heart condition, and she developed cancer. I did not want to follow in her health footsteps.

I was a caregiver for my mother for three years. I saw her problems on a day-to-day basis, as well as in and out of the hospital. Believe me, you *want* to do everything possible to stay out of the hospital. I think most of you know what I mean. It is not going to get any better.

III. THINGS I LEARNED (AND CONTINUE TO LEARN) FROM MY FATHER

The things I remember most about my father during my growing up years are his hard work, his honesty, his integrity, and his quietness in comparison to my mother. My father worked outdoors for most of his life, handled hard physical labor, worked long hours, and never complained. I have never heard him say a negative word about anyone. My mother ran the household. My father silently consented. I never really got to know my father when I was growing up.

My father is now ninety-four years old, lives by himself and his four-year-old dog, Buddy. He is in good health. Almost every day he swims, bicycles, and gardens in his yard. He takes Buddy on long walks. He reads the paper daily, he watches the news, and all shapes and sizes of sporting events on television. He discusses current events with me—he keeps an active mind. He and I have taken nine cruises together since my mother died four years ago.

Last summer I took my father back to our hometown to see some of his old friends. When you are ninety-four you do not have too many old friends left. We saw five or six of his friends. All were recuperating from fractures.

Now that people are living longer, we adult children are increasingly handling a new job: being caregivers for our parents. It's said that one reason for being kind to your children as you raise them, if for no other reason, is because they are the ones who may eventually select your nursing home. Notwithstanding, if our parents can maintain good health as they age, the nursing home option can be deferred, perhaps indefinitely. The caregiver job is crucial, demanding, and rewarding.

The most rewarding part of caring for my father is that I have finally gotten to really know him. I visit him every day. I make him dinner. We shop. We go on errands. We hang out together. His wonderful attitude sustains not only him, but also sustains me.

IV. THINGS I LEARNED FROM (OR TAUGHT TO) MY HUSBAND

Play the Odds: Younger MAN, Older WOMAN!

Women typically live longer then men. Why? My husband delights in telling me that husbands usually die before wives, because they want to. But it is sad to say that men's lifestyle choices play a major role in increasing their risks for both disability and premature death. We know that compared to women, men tend to: eat more fat, eat less vegetables, eat less fruit, drink, smoke, use more recreational drugs, engage in riskier behavior, get less sleep, visit doctors less often, be less likely to follow doctors' instructions, and get less regular exercise.

In a typical marriage, why is the husband older than the wife? Is there any cosmic logic to such an age arrangement? Men typically live a shorter life-span than women. Giving the husband a head start in the age race doesn't make a lot of biological sense. In my first marriage, my husband was eight years older. He was set in his ways when we married—I had to adapt. I took five years trying to land him—I took twelve years trying to get rid of him.

I took a different approach in my second marriage. When we met in 1980, I was forty-one years old while Jim was just twenty-nine. I was a single parent with a precocious six-year-old son, working as the new home sales director in a waterfront development. Even though Jim seemed like a nice guy, I complained to the girls at the office that he was too young, and nothing like what I was looking for. I was looking for a mature, older man...with money! The girls in the office said, "He really has potential, he's a nice guy, he has no 'baggage.' Best of all, you can mold him into whatever you want him to be." I reflected on what they said, and decided he might be a keeper. The "molding" part really appealed to me.

Jim was a lawyer who was brought in to tell fifteen of my buyers that the development couldn't build their homes for the contract price, and that they should take their deposits back. I lost fifteen sales commissions, but gained a husband! He likes to tell people I'm still not sure whether I got a good deal. He was right, I didn't get a *good* deal—I got the *deal of a lifetime*! Ladies, go younger. I highly recommend it!

Laughter is a Magic Pill

We've been married twenty-five years. My husband is still my best friend; he still makes me laugh, often and loud–chuckles, guffaws, belly laughs–all shapes and sizes. Surveys of women consistently show that the most important characteristic women look for in a man is a good sense of humor—someone to make them laugh.

In an earlier generation, Norman Cousins' story of how he employed humor to recover from a life-threatening illness was well known. Norman Cousins was the editor of the *Saturday Review* magazine for almost forty years, among other notable things. In the 1960s he developed a life-threatening disease. Part of his treatment was a daily dose of positive emotions, including belly laughter from watching classic comedy movies. His book, *Anatomy of an Illness as Perceived by the Patient*, was published in 1979 and is still readily available.

Subsequent studies suggest that laughter and happiness tend to:

- Boost the immune system;
- Lessen pain;
- Reduce stress;
- Increase the ability to cope with problems;
- Lead to better marriages; and
- Lead to higher self-esteem.

A good laugh is good for the body and good for the soul. Children laugh hundreds of times a day, adults just a few. Try to be more child-like—try to see humor in many situations. It's the healthy and fun thing to do. It can also be a fashion tip—the best thing to wear is a big smile.

Human Molting

I was able to do a lot of molding of Jim, and the process will almost certainly never end. I think that this process may be one important aspect of the marital relationship. However, it doesn't go only one way—Jim has also helped mold me. I don't consider it just "molding" any more. I now think of it as being a process of human "molting"—developing in a positive direction.

Jim never smoked, so I was not tempted to start smoking again. He never drank alcohol, and he was able to help me quit in 1989. He convinced me that a tan wasn't beautiful; rather it was the result of burst blood vessels in the skin. I stopped sun bathing. I started wearing sunscreen when I planned to go out in the sun. He got me out to start playing tennis and golf again. He adopted my son, and has always been a full partner in raising our son. He generally has helped me live a healthier life.

A few years ago when I decided to quit real estate, I didn't know what I wanted to do next. I was reading what he refers to as "trash" novels every night. He encouraged (more accurately "challenged") me to read something more constructive, something that could increase my knowledge or have a greater benefit for me. So on a nightly basis I started reading and studying materials on health and fitness. My life took a turn in its present direction. I continue to study health and fitness, and to apply my knowledge to my own life. This has also led me to try to help others through my speaking and writing. My efforts have come full circle, even helping Jim, who helped start me on this road.

Periodic Checkups and Colonoscopies

Like the shoemaker's child who goes shoeless, and the attorney's family having no wills, bright people don't always take simple steps to check their health. Most men take care of their cars better than they take care of themselves. They check the oil and tune up their car engines; but they don't have periodic checkups of their bodies. They're also raised with the mentality to ignore pain. Some also go through life ignoring symptoms, believing that if they ignore a problem long enough, it will go away.

Katie Couric, the *Today Show* host, publicized the colonoscopy procedure a few years ago, by having her own colonoscopy done live on national television. Her husband, Jay Monahan, had died of colon cancer that had been undetected until symptoms appeared. Cancer of the colon can develop for many years before any symptoms appear. Like high blood pressure, it can be a silent killer. Estimates are that more than 150,000 people will be diagnosed this year with colon cancer in our country alone. Colon cancer is the second leading cause of cancer death in our country.

A colonoscopy is a procedure in which a camera is used to check the colon for cancer or for polyps. As part of the procedure, small polyps can be removed. The procedure is not as cumbersome or uncomfortable as it had been a few years ago. You now drink clear liquids with a small amount of solution the day before, to clean your system. The day of the colonoscopy, you go to a doctor's office or a hospital as an outpatient; you are put under general anesthesia and the next thing you know, you are finished. The procedure usually takes about thirty minutes and is painless. My husband and I were having lunch together two hours after we had ours done.

I spoke to my husband Jim four years ago (when he became fifty) about having a colonoscopy, to check for colon cancer or precancerous polyps. He seemed to always have a reason to put it off. Two years ago, he finally agreed to have the procedure, if I would also have a colonoscopy. It is sometimes true that there is nothing like "togetherness"—we each had a colonoscopy. My results were fine. Jim had a problem—he had a polyp too large to be removed as part of the colonoscopy procedure.

Jim was referred to a surgeon for removal of a portion of his colon. The operation was done using the newer technique known as laparoscopic surgery. Instead of long, deep cuts through the abdomen wall, a minimally invasive series of small incisions is made in the abdomen. A small video camera is placed through one of the incisions, allowing the surgeon a magnified view of the patient's internal organs. Surgical instruments are placed through the other incisions. Generally laparoscopic surgery, compared to traditional open surgery, involves less pain, quicker recovery, and a shorter hospital stay. The National Institute of Health conducted a study published in the *New England Journal of Medicine* in 2004, indicating that laparoscopic surgery is as effective as traditional open surgery in treating colon cancer. Jim was out of the hospital in four days. He was the chair and moderator of a seminar for 450 lawyers less than fourteen days after the operation.

Jim's surgeon said the operation was totally successful. The bonus, he joked, was that the next time Jim has a colonoscopy, he will only be charged three quarters of the regular fee, because there will be less colon to search. I hope that Jim's success story will encourage those of you and your family who are fifty years of age or older, or those who have a family history of colon cancer, to have a colonoscopy.

Jim's story was part of the success story of the "Couric Effect," the increase in colon cancer screenings directly related to Katie Couric. Jim and I owe her an immeasurable debt. The Jay Monahan Center for Gastrointestinal Health opened its doors on March 30, 2004. Named in honor of Katie's husband, it is a clinical center of the New York Presbyterian Hospital and the Weill Cornell Medical College. For information about the center, about gastrointestinal health, or to be placed on an information mailing list, visit the web site: http://www.monahancenter.org.

Gentlemen, listen to your wives, not just about getting a colonoscopy, but about getting checkups in general. Wives usually live longer than you men do; they want *you* to live longer too. Listen to your partner—learn from one another.

Sex Is Not Just for the Chronologically Young

What are the side effects of good health? One side effect is looking good—even years younger. An Arabian proverb sums it up: "He who hath good health is young." Although we may believe it ought not be this way, physical appearance can be an important plus in the competitive world of finding a partner. Getting in shape has its benefits: looking good, being fit, being healthy and, yes, attracting the opposite sex.

Sex is a part of us until our dying days. Granted, the quality and quantity may vary. I recently repeated a joke to a group of older women, about more money being spent on Viagra and breast implants than on Alzheimer's research. The punch line was we will end up with an elderly population with perky boobs and erections, but not remembering what to do with them. A nurse who cares for Alzheimer's patients chimed in to correct me: "Oh yes they do!"

Sexual vitality can keep you young. A great sex life can even make you feel and look younger. A general rule of thumb says that three times a week can make you ten years younger. I don't think this means that nine times a week can make you thirty years younger. But safe, regular sexual activity itself is also a big factor in maintaining sexual health, and health in general. It is the old concept of "use it or lose it." Not only can it make you younger, it can ease stress, improve sleep, and leave you with an overall deeper sense of well-being. By adhering to a healthy lifestyle and boosting your sexual vitality, you can continue to feel frisky throughout your golden years. There is no reason you can't be:

- Fabulous at fifty,
- Sexy at sixty,
- Sensational at seventy,
- Energetic at eighty, and even
- Naughty at ninety.

Women and men who take care of their general health are usually the sexiest and the most sexually active. I have listened to Dr. Ruth speak at two AARP conventions. She keeps her audiences giggling like teenagers. Dr. Ruth has published several informative books, my favorite being *Sex for Dummies*. It is never too late for a refresher course.

Yes, I married a younger man, but in spite of his relative youth, he is still able to keep up with me.

V. THINGS I LEARNED FROM MY DOGS

We were having breakfast on a Saturday. I was reading the Boca paper, and saw an advertisement by the local Humane Society that said, "Special sale on dogs, this weekend only." "Why don't we take a look at the animal shelter after breakfast?" I asked my husband. "I think a dog would be a good companion for my father." My mother had died a few months earlier. My ninety-year-old father was now living alone.

"Is this a ploy for us to get another dog?" my husband asked— our dog had died two years earlier. We had decided not to replace our dog because of our busy schedules.

"No," I assured him, "this is to get a dog to be company for my father."

We finished breakfast and went to the shelter. When we arrived, I immediately settled on two puppies in a pen just inside the door. Inside the pen was also a very strange looking dog standing on top of a cage barking. This strange-looking dog had her fur clipped short, overly long ears, and tiny teeth with an under bite. She looked more like a gremlin than a dog. She cocked her head as she looked at each person coming through the door with her one eye. I asked the first person I met what we needed to do to adopt one of the puppies.

I was told that there was a long waiting list for the puppies. They asked us to look at the other dogs to see if we might want to adopt one of them. We looked through the kennels, but my heart was set on one of the puppies. I spoke to the shelter person again and explained that I was only interested in a puppy. After a short interview session, reviewing our history of having dogs for forty years, we were told to wait in the other room.

We sat at a table. In came the director of the shelter with some paperwork. She reviewed the paperwork with us and as we were about to finalize the puppy adoption, she said, "it would really be wonderful if you could also adopt the puppy's mother—she's been abused and with only one eye, we think she will not be adoptable." To my amazement, I heard this voice immediately say "we would love to." My husband the softie said this spontaneously, without hesitation or discussion.

We named the puppy "Buddy." Buddy went to live with my father, where he has been a faithful, constant companion. We keep Mandy at our house. Mandy is a Cairn Terrier mix—like "Toto" in the Wizard of Oz movie.

Mandy's fur has grown back in thick and fluffy. Barely a day goes by without someone on the street commenting "What a cute dog—what kind is it?" We think of her as a heart wrapped in fur.

We recently adopted a third Humane Society dog, Annie. Annie has the sweetest disposition imaginable. She looks like the movie dog "Benji." She can be handled as if she were a rag doll. Annie and Mandy are now therapy dogs. I take them to various nursing homes, health facilities, and speaking functions where they bring as much joy to others as they continue to bring to my husband and to me. Annie loves to give kisses to everyone, which are warmly welcomed. Mandy seems to speak in her own language to people when she greets them. Things could not have worked out better for all concerned.

Health Benefits of Having a Pet

According to the National Institutes of Health, animals as pets have played a significant role in human history. Keeping pets was common in hunter-gathering societies. For centuries, horseback riding has been used for people with serious disabilities. Animals were incorporated into the treatment for mental patients in England in 1792. Dogs were used in 1919 in this country as companions for resident patients in psychiatric hospitals. The great increase in pet ownership today perhaps reflects an unsatisfied need for intimacy, nurturing, and contact with nature. There is evidence of a correlation between pet ownership and pet attachment in combating depression. Animal visitation programs to nursing homes can lead older people to smile more, talk more, reach out, exhibit more alertness, and experience symptoms of well-being and less depression.

According to the National Center for Infectious Diseases, the majority of American households have at least one pet. Having a pet can:

- Decrease your blood pressure;
- Decrease cholesterol levels;
- Decrease triglyceride levels;
- Decrease feelings of loneliness;
- Increase opportunities for exercise;
- Increase opportunities for outdoor activities, and
- Increase opportunities for socialization.

There are many other studies regarding healthy reasons to have a pet. In addition to those benefits listed above by the National Center for Infectious Diseases, the benefits of having a pet (or a pet visitor) can include:

- Higher level of activities of daily living for seniors;
- Coping better with stress;
- Fewer minor health problems;
- Lower medication costs for persons in nursing home facilities;
- Better physical health due to exercise with a pet; and
- Increased family happiness.

Therapy Dogs

A dog is not concerned with age or physical ability. A dog accepts people as they are. In addition to the health benefits discussed above, a therapy dog visiting a health care facility can offer entertainment and a welcome distraction from pain or infirmity. The visit from a therapy dog can provide a welcome change from routine. Periodic visits can provide something to look forward to. Petting a dog can reduce blood pressure; it encourages stretching, turning, and use of hands and arms. A pet gives two strangers something in common, making it easier for them to talk. These benefits can continue after the visit ends, leaving memories and anticipation of future visits. Annie and Mandy give joy to everyone they've visited. Do you have a dog that might bring joy into the lives of the disabled or elderly simply by visiting them?

VI. THINGS I LEARNED FROM MYSELF

Smoking and drinking used to be very commonly accepted—what many people enjoyed. I can remember as a stewardess handing out cigarettes, compliments of the RJ Reynolds Tobacco Company. I also remember champagne flowing while I served filet mignon. Boy, have those "coffee, tea or me" days of flying changed!

Menopause and Osteoporosis

My problem started about twelve years ago–about the time of the "M" word. "Menopause" is a word that conjures up images of an aging body, a wrinkled body, and an end of youth and attractiveness. Just before we go into menopause, our bodies start changing. Metabolism really slows down.

When I "reached" the age of fifty-one, I met the Seven Dwarfs of Menopause described by Suzanne Somers: Itchy, Bitchy, Sweaty, Sleepy, Bloated, Forgetful, and All-Dried-Up. I decided to do something about this uninvited gang.

At the age of fifty-two—a year after starting to deal with those Seven Dwarfs—I had my first bone density test. I found I had osteoporosis. Having been active in sports and working out my entire life, I was surprised. I grew up in Wisconsin, eating lots of dairy and good food. What had I done wrong? I smoked starting in my teenage years until the age of thirty-eight. I also drank alcohol–certainly *not* in moderation, and I loved coffee *with* caffeine. Smoking, alcohol, and caffeine will rob our bones of calcium leaving them brittle and subject to fracture.

It is not normal for us to get shorter and more fragile when we age. However, this happens much too often. Woman—especially those with small frames—who do not exercise are more prone to develop osteoporosis. Men are less likely to develop the disease until they reach seventy-five, when men and women are equally likely to develop the crippling disease—a disease which causes one half of our elderly population to lose their independence due to one or more fractures.

At fifty-two I had become overweight. I was diagnosed with severe osteoporosis of the hip. It was time to get serious about my health or suffer all the health problems my Mother had. Osteoporosis is a medical condition in which the bones become brittle and fragile–typically as a result of hormonal changes, or deficiency of calcium or vitamin D. It is preventable and reversible. What did I do to improve my condition? I took off the weight—fifty pounds of it. I joined a gym and worked with a trainer to learn the correct way to use weights. I worked out with weight machines three times a week. I started eating a healthy, calcium-rich diet. I totally reversed my condition. I schedule a bone scan every few years to monitor my bone density.

It is never too early to take care of our bones. They are an element of staying healthy that will keep us independent in our later years. So many aging people have fractures—it is a widespread problem with people as they age. So remember: be tested, eat calcium-rich food, exercise, including some type of weight bearing exercise and stay away from calcium robbers: alcohol and caffeine.

Make sure you get your mammogram, too. I recently saw an e-mail telling young women how to prepare for their first mammogram. The email suggested inviting a friend over to help you. Go to your kitchen, open your refrigerator door, insert one breast between the door and the frame, and ask your friend to slam the door shut, and lean on the door for good measure, hold that position for five seconds while you hold your breath, then repeat on the other side. ONLY KIDDING!

Today, both the bone density test and the mammogram tests are very quick and painless. My first bone density test took about thirty minutes lying flat on a cold metal table with a slow-moving machine going over me. Today it usually takes less than five minutes.

I no longer drink alcoholic beverages. I also stopped smoking more than thirty years ago. In the past forty years, the U.S. Surgeon General has issued twenty-eight reports on smoking. The first was issued in 1964. It concluded that cigarette smoking was a cause of lung cancer and laryngeal cancer in men, a probable cause of lung cancer in women, and the most important cause of chronic bronchitis. The 2004 report (which is 960 pages long) contains an Executive Summary with Table 1.1 that finds a causal relationship between smoking and the following:

- Cancers:
Bladder cancer, cervical cancer, esophageal cancer, kidney cancer, laryngeal cancer, leukemia, lung cancer, oral cancer, pancreatic cancer, and stomach cancer;

- Cardiovascular Diseases:
Abdominal aortic aneurysm, arteriosclerosis, cerebrovascular disease, coronary heart disease;

- Respiratory Diseases:
Chronic obstructive pulmonary disease; pneumonia; respiratory effects in utero (reduced lung function in infants), respiratory effects in childhood and adolescence (impaired lung growth during childhood and adolescence, early onset of lung function decline, asthma-related symptoms, coughing, phlegm, wheezing, and dyspnea), respiratory effects in adulthood (premature onset and accelerated age-related decline in lung function, coughing, phlegm, wheezing, and dyspnea, and poor asthma control);

- Reproductive Effects:
Fetal death and stillbirths, fertility, low birth weight, pregnancy complications;

- Other Effects:
Cataracts, diminished health status/morbidity, hip fractures, low bone density, and peptic ulcer.

There is very little in the body that is not negatively affected by cigarette smoke. One conclusion of the report which gives me hope (since I haven't smoked in thirty years) is that there is a connection between "sustained cessation from smoking" and a return of the rate of decline in pulmonary function to those of a person who has never smoked. I should breathe easier. Stop smoking now, and maybe you will too.

Exercising Doesn't Have to be as Excruciating as an Exorcism

Exercise is critical for good health and a longer life. Exercise helps you lose excess weight or maintain a proper weight by burning fat and increasing muscle tissue. Exercise can improve digestion, improve sleep, lower blood pressure, improve cholesterol levels, increase mental alertness, strengthen muscles, strengthen bones, increase flexibility, improve stamina, reduce depression, and improve self-esteem. Exercise can reduce anxiety, reduce stress, help maintain healthy sexual relations, decrease the risk of heart disease, and lower the risk of certain cancers.

How is exercise like the weather? A quotation often attributed to Mark Twain says, "Everybody talks about the weather, but nobody does anything about it." As a nation it seems everyone talks about exercise, but the great majority of us do nothing about it. Why do we continue to be a nation of couch potatoes when we know better?

In a survey of adults we find people are more afraid of public speaking than of dying. The comedian's punch line is that most people who attend a funeral would rather be in the coffin than giving the eulogy. Exercise runs close behind death and public speaking as far as an activity to be avoided. Why don't people exercise? Why is there an apparent epidemic of fitness phobia?

Physical fitness became a material concern of our federal government at least as early as 1953 with a negative report about the physical fitness of American children relative to European children. In 1956 President Eisenhower created the President's Council on Youth Fitness, with cabinet-level status. The objective of the Council was to create public awareness of the importance of physical fitness and how to improve it. President Kennedy changed the original name of the Council to the President's Council on Physical Fitness to include all ages. He also launched a public service advertising campaign. State centers were established to demonstrate model elementary and secondary school programs. President Johnson changed the Council's name to the President's Council on Physical Fitness and Sports. An objective was to encourage continuing fitness through sports and games. The attention of the federal government has continued and evolved under the Nixon, Ford, Carter, Bush, Clinton, and Bush administrations. On June 16, 2004, the Healthier U.S. Fitness

Festival was held on the National Mall in Washington, D.C., with the Congressional Fitness Caucus. A web site has been established at www.presidentschallenge.org to provide basic information by age group for activities to improve physical fitness.

For those of you who saw the movie *The Exorcist* you know that exorcizing a demon is not pleasant, to say the least—the fight between good and evil usually is hard. The fight against bad health need not be so excruciatingly painful if you follow a few simple rules.

First, choose an exercise. It might be aerobics or bicycling or cheerleading or dancing or golf or jogging or walking or one of a hundred other activities. One of the easiest forms of exercise is walking. Walking burns almost as many calories as jogging, swimming or aerobics classes.

If you want some ideas, go to the www.presidentschallenge.org web site.

Second, be sure the exercise is something you enjoy. If you don't like it, you won't do it; if you don't do it, it won't benefit you.

Third, exercise for thirty minutes a day, five days a week. Of course this can vary by age group, by the nature of the activity, and by the person's particular health condition and circumstances.

Fourth, keep a log of your activity. The key is to find something you really enjoy doing and then get into the habit of doing it—make a standing date with yourself.

That's it. Certainly nothing to make your head spin!

Diet Versus Dieting

Dieting—the dreaded "D" word. Diets come, diets go. Fad diets will probably always be popular, even more popular as more and more of us get larger and larger. Beware of diets that exclude any of the basic food groups—excluding any of the food groups can do harm to the body's cells.

As a nation we are the fattest on the globe. Just look around, or perhaps just look in the mirror. It just seems harder and harder to keep the physique we once had, or to obtain the physique we desire.

The American lifestyle continues to contribute to the problem. Our busy lives are stressful. We eat to make us feel better about problems. We eat on the run. We are categorically impatient. We demand immediate foods, not just fast foods. We trade a lot in exchange for convenience. The idea of eating three home-cooked, properly balanced meals per day has become a relic of our history.

In the past forty years the average weight for an American man has increased from about 165 pounds to about 190 pounds. The average weight for an American woman has increased by about twenty-five pounds. The average weight for an American child has increased by more than ten pounds.

There is a problem with both the quality and the quantity of what we eat. This brings to mind the conversation between two women at a restaurant. One remarks that the food is not very good. The other, while agreeing, goes on to complain, "And the portions aren't large, either."

This year is the fiftieth anniversary of McDonald's. There are more than 31,000 McDonald's restaurants in more than 100 countries around the world. Last year when we vacationed in Germany we saw a seemingly countless number of McDonald's signs dotting the Autobahn, even near tiny towns. Last year a movie titled "Supersize Me" chronicled McDonald's. The movie, in a modified form, is being shown in health classes in our high schools to make young adults aware of the hazards they deal with regarding fast food. This movie is a must see for you. We do not need "supersized" food. There is nothing super about it—what ultimately gets "supersized" is us. Most restaurants—not just McDonald's—serve portions that are just too large. Sometimes we don't know if the restaurant name is describing the food they serve or the people they want to create—take Blimpie's for example.

The fast food phenomenon—particularly its marketing—has had the effect of programming children to demand they eat at their favorite fast food restaurants. The fact that our children are learning the fast food habit may be the nutrition tragedy of our lifetime. We are raising children who will become ticking health time bombs at a very early age. Forty million American children have abnormally high cholesterol levels. By age twelve, it is estimated that seventy percent have the beginning stages of arteriosclerosis—hardening of the arteries. We are in danger of becoming the first generation where some of us can expect to outlive our children. Health problems and the cost of health care will continue to spiral upward. The statistics on heart problems, diabetes, and many related health problems that come from being obese will continue to increase exponentially.

In addition to the quantity of the food we eat, the quality continues to deteriorate. Fast foods are loaded with fats, sugar, salt, and preservatives. Some studies show that eating just fifty grams of fat at one sitting can cause arteries to begin deteriorating. Beyond fast foods, food manufacturers throughout the years—the last fifty years—have changed the way they make our food. I'm talking about processed foods and enriched flours. Whole grains that are so healthy for us are being ground into a fine powdery substance—enriched flour products—devoid of most of their original natural nutrients and made into our breads, cereals, crackers, and pastas. When consumed, it turns into a sugary substance and, if not burned up, is stored in our bodies as fat. It takes a lot of energy to burn all the excess sugar our bodies are getting.

We need to read labels. We need to eat whole grains and whole wheats. Bubbling hydrogen gas through vegetable oil, a process called "hydrogenation," creates trans fats. Trans fats can clog arteries and lurk in a multitude of foods. Manufacturers do not label the amount of trans fats, and will not by law until 2006. Food manufacturers use the hydrogenation process to give products longer shelf life. It's hard to find true whole wheat bread at the supermarkets. Read the label carefully before you conclude that what is marked as "whole wheat" is actually 100 percent whole wheat.

When I was a child, many foods were not only healthier but they tasted better. I remember growing vegetables in our garden, picking them fresh, and eating them without having them processed, frozen, or stored. Fruits and vegetables from our supermarkets contain much less nutrition than if they were homegrown. Most are not vine ripened, sit in storage, and are a month or so old before we get them.

I dine out more often than I should. My main defense is to take half of my meal home. I also stay away from breads, sauces, and fatty salad dressings. I also stay away from sugar and caffeine. I avoid fried foods, and I totally abstain from fried foods prepared by a process which re-uses oil. The more the oil is used, the worse for your health.

I drink plenty of water and green tea. Water is a bona fide miracle—it is the greatest nutritional supplement in the world. If you don't drink an adequate amount of water, you are liable to find it impossible to achieve control over your weight and your health. Some suggest ten twelve-ounce glasses of water daily. Other fluids don't count.

The last time I returned to my old high school for a class reunion I was appalled to see that the cafeteria no longer served hot lunches. The walls of the cafeteria were lined with vending machines. Do you know whether this is happening in your schools?

The U.S. Department of Health and Human Services and U.S. Department of Agriculture are mandated to revise and issue Dietary Guidelines for Americans. *The Dietary Guidelines for Americans 2005* (http://www.health.gov/dietaryguidelines/dga2005/report/) summarize and synthesize knowledge about individual nutrients and food components into recommendations for a pattern of eating for the public. Two examples of such eating patterns that exemplify the *Dietary Guidelines for Americans 2005* are the *USDA Food Guide* (http://www.usda.gov/cnpp/pyramid.html) and the *DASH (Dietary Approaches to Stop Hypertension) Eating Plan* (http://www.nhlbi.nih.gov/health/public/heart/hbp/dash/). These eating patterns are not weight loss diets.

Some of the recommendations from the *Dietary Guidelines for Americans 2005* include:

1. Consume a variety of nutrient-dense foods and beverages among the basic food groups.
2. Limit the intake of saturated and trans fats, cholesterol, sugars, salt, and alcohol.
3. Adopt a balanced eating pattern.
4. Engage in regular physical activity *and* reduce sedentary activities.
5. Achieve physical fitness by cardiovascular conditioning, stretching for flexibility, and resistance exercises or calisthenics for muscle strength.
6. Consume a sufficient amount of fiber-rich fruits and vegetables, and whole-grain products.
7. For those who drink alcoholic beverages, do so in moderation (defined as up to one drink a day for women, up to two drinks per day for men). Alcohol should not be consumed by some individuals (e.g., people who can't restrict their alcohol intake, pregnant and lactating women, individuals taking

medications that can interact with alcohol, and people with certain medical conditions).

Some nutritionists criticize the *Daily Guidelines* for failing to state clearly, "eat less," and to adequately warn against salt, saturated fat, and cholesterol.

Health and Wealth

Our society is preoccupied with accumulating wealth. Without health, however, wealth doesn't really matter. This is not an earth-shaking revelation, hot off the press. Quotations through-out the centuries observe this most important connection:

"Health without money is half an ague."
[An "ague" is a chill or a fit of shivering.]

"The first wealth is health."

"Nor love, nor honour, wealth nor power, can give the heart a cheerful hour when health is lost."

"If all be well with belly, feet, and sides, a king's estate no greater good provides."

"Life is not merely to be alive, but to be well."

"Without health, life is not life; life is lifeless."

"All health is better than wealth."

"Oh blessed health...He that has thee, has little more to wish for; and he that is so wretched as to want thee, wants everything with thee."

"Ask me no more which is the greatest wealth, our rich possessions, liberty or health."

Some things just go together—salt and pepper, yin and yang, and wealth and health. The words "wealth" and "health" do more than just rhyme. They complement each other. We all know many people with material wealth who would gladly exchange their material wealth for good health. You can't enjoy wealth, without good health. For most people, health is not valued until sickness comes. Choose health now. Choose health over wealth if you must choose.

It IS Better to Give Than to Receive

We've all heard it many times in various paraphrased forms: "It is better to give than to receive" (Acts 20:35). A variation is that "In giving, a man receives more than he gives, and the more is in proportion to the worth of the thing given."

I am a volunteer speaker for the National Osteoporosis Foundation. I am certified as a colon cancer educator, as well as a nutrition and physical activity educator, for the American Cancer Society. I am a member of the Board of the American Health Association, which is a Boca Raton-based charity with a major emphasis on preventive health. I love volunteering for the various American Health Association campaigns during the holidays. "Santa Cause I Love You" involves the heartwarming experience of delivering teddy bears to patients in various facilities (i.e., nursing, assisted living, rehabilitation, wellness), as well as to children in childcare centers for the needy. My therapy dogs accompany me in delivering the teddy bears, wearing their Santa or elf hats, and bring even more joy. Sometimes my dogs are mistaken for stuffed animals. The Association is presently also involved in sending 50,000 stuffed animals to orphans in Iraq.

Research shows people who are giving appear to live longer. Dr. Wayne Dyer has observed that through giving and through other acts of kindness our immune systems are strengthened and our seratonin levels are increased. Serve your community as a volunteer. There are so many non-profit organizations needing help. Find one that shares your interests and your passions, or identify what you are good at. Few things are as rewarding as the giving of yourself. Teaching, gardening, accounting, painting, cooking, organizing, cleaning, driving, being a companion—there is a volunteer position out there waiting just for you. Volunteering will not only keep your mind and body stimulated and energized, it will help those in need. It *is* better to give than to receive, because in the act of giving to others, *you* also receive.

A Summary of Some General Suggestions

We can summarize some general health suggestions as follows:

1. Take responsibility for your health. Listen to your body. Schedule yearly physicals.
2. Get involved. Enjoy a good social life. Develop a network of friends. Have a spiritual life. Find your passions and purposes in your life. Help others. Volunteer.
3. Keep physically and mentally active. Keep learning. Take up a hobby. Take up a sport. Keep exercising. Make such activities life-long habits.
4. Simplify your life. Keep it less stressful. Keep it simple, less cluttered.
5. Laugh and develop your sense of humor. There is power in laughter. Be a child again. Children laugh hundreds of times a day, adults only a few. Laugh. Laugh at yourself. Make someone else laugh. It's the healthy thing to do.
6. Bad things will happen in life. When they do, grieve, endure, and then get on with your life.
7. Surround yourself with love, happiness, friends, family, and a pet. Love them. Regularly tell them you love them.
8. Cherish your health. If it is good, preserve it. If it is not good, improve it. If you need help, get help.

VII. CONCLUSION

I have titled this chapter "Looking Good and Feeling Good at any Age: Some Things I have Learned so Far." I hope to do a lot more living and a lot more learning. In the interim, I recommend the following prayer to help you end each day:

A Prayer to End the Day (Anonymous)

> *NOW I lay me down to SLEEP,*
> *I pray the LORD my shape to keep,*
> *Please no WRINKLES,*
> *Please no BAGS,*
> *Lift my BUTT*
> *Before it SAGS.*
> *Please no AGE SPOTS,*
> *Please no GRAY,*
> *As for my BELLY, take it AWAY.*
> *Keep me HEALTHY,*
> *Keep me YOUNG,*
> *AND THANK YOU LORD*
> *For all you've DONE.*

These are some of the things I have learned so far. I invite you to join me in this lifelong learning process.

About The Author

Gwen Herb

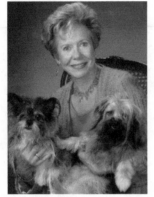

Gwen Herb has developed a speaking program "Looking Good and Feeling Great at Any Age." Her speeches are designed to give her audience ideas to improve the quality of their lives through healthy diet and fitness routines. Gwen emphasizes prevention and precautions before problems arise. She is a member of the Florida Speakers Association and the National Speakers Association. She has achieved the competent leader and advanced toastmaster designations from Toastmasters International. She has spoken on behalf of the National Osteoporosis Foundation, as well as on behalf of the National Cancer Association, for which she is certified to speak as a colon cancer educator and a nutrition and physical activity educator. She is a member of the board of the American Health Association, a charity devoted to preventive health. She is president of Gwen Herb Smart Health, Inc., her own corporation committed to promoting health and fitness. Her chapter reduces to writing some of her thoughts and experiences about health and aging.

Gwen Herb
Gwen Herb Smart Health, Inc.
2200 Corp. Blvd. N.W., Suite 317
Boca Raton, FL 33431
Phone: 561.487.1218
Fax: 561.982.9934
E-mail: ggherb1@aol.com
Web: www.gwenherbsmarthealth.com

Chapter 8

It's Your Movie™
Seeing Life through a Female Lens

Carolyn Strauss

Concept: How's the movie? You ask, "what movie?" It's the movie of your life. In other words, *your life* is *your movie.*

Most of us are too close to our own lives to have the perspective to see what is actually there, or more importantly, make changes for ourselves. Change is always difficult and sometimes painful. Even positive change can be unsettling to us and to those around us. So, what if we look at life as a personal movie? *You* are the director, the producer, the star, the writer, and even the casting agent. You decide who comes in, who goes out, what your motivation is at any time, and if something is not going according to "script" or plan, you have the power to change it.

The following chapter is an excerpt from a speech I gave to 200 women at a "Women in Business" breakfast. Imagine you are there, get yourself some coffee, sit back and enjoy. And thank you for your time—I believe time is your most precious resource. Always spend yours on what matters.

Premise: Women have come remarkably far in the past fifty years. Any woman between the age of twenty and fifty-four was told either directly or subtly that she could do anything a man could do, she could do it better, she could do it faster, she could do it smarter, and she could probably handle it all even more competently. She was told that she should be paid the same amount of money for it as a man (which makes perfect sense). Our fore-mothers—women who went out into the world to do this, women who are now in their forties, fifties and sixties—forged their way into the workplace so that future generations of women could have the careers they wanted. When they went into the work-force, they had no role models who were doing "work" in a feminine way—working in a feminine paradigm. So, these "trail-blazers" went out and looked at who was successful in business: Men. They modeled themselves after men in the workplace. Men were and are successful in the workplace for several reasons I'll get to in a moment. But first, let's start with three basic assump-tions that seem universal, based on the thousands of women I've spoken with all across the country:

Assumptions:

1.   Every woman has personal and professional goals she's working toward achieving.
2.   Every woman gives 100 percent of herself in every area of her life whenever possible.
3.   Every woman reading this is generally exhausted, depleted, drained and needs a vacation.

The masculine paradigm: All of this stems from approach-ing our lives from a masculine paradigm. There are several components of the masculine paradigm:

Single focus: Men are single-focused. Have you ever walked into a room when there was a man watching television, you try to talk with him and he's completely ignoring you? I have some good news—he's not ignoring you. A man cannot be watching television *and* ignoring you. He's just watching television. He does one thing at a time and he generally does that very well. Here's why: If we look back in time to the days when we lived in caves, the man's job was to go out into the world and hunt for food. They had to "hunt the deer." Men were out with a single focus—"hunting the deer." If they were like women, and multi-tasked they would be "hunting the deer" until they found a pretty flower. (Deer's gone. Oops!) Men are genetically programmed to "hunt the deer,"—to be single-focused—because if they didn't, women didn't eat, and the species would die off.

Competition: Men are also biologically competitive—it is in their nature to be competitive. After man hunted the deer, man had to kill it. (Luckily women didn't have to do that.) Men had to compete with other men all the time in order to provide for themselves and their family. They had to focus, they had to kill, and they had to fight to get the deer for their family.

Multi-tasking: Biologically, women multi-task. Back to the cave person days: women were taking care of the cave, making babies, and feeding the babies. Women were cleaning, cooking the food, and feeding the hunter. Women made everything okay by taking care of everything at the same time. In modern times, when women went out into the work force, we became more single-focused and more competitive in order to succeed and survive in a man's world.

Testosterone: Do you know where that single-focus, and the ability to kill comes from in men? It comes from testosterone. Men have the biological facility to produce testosterone in their testicles.

Where does testosterone come from in women? Women's bodies biologically produce testosterone in the adrenal glands. Today women's adrenal glands are working harder than they've ever worked. Women's bodies are producing more adrenaline and more testosterone than ever before.

Illness: After studying this, I have developed a theory: Many women are having trouble conceiving, and are getting stress-related illnesses because of all the testosterone in their bodies and how hard their adrenal glands are working. It's just a theory.

So women are biologically multi-tasking but working and living in this competitive, single-focused masculine paradigm.

Demonstration: While reading this, imagine your life and fill in the details as they apply to you.

The alarm clock rings, you wake up in the morning. How many of us thought when the alarm clock rang this morning, "Aaah, good! What a nice calm happy morning feeling? I can lay here. I can snooze for ten minutes. Mmmm great! What a nice day I am going to have at this breakfast meeting at 7:30—it'll be fun. I am all relaxed." Or did your alarm clock ring and it was panic, "Oh my God! It's already 5:30! I've got to get up! I've got to get out of bed!" You jump out of bed with your heart pounding. How many of us start our day with our heart racing like crazy? You start our day by jumping into the shower, and while in the shower, thinking about the twenty or thirty things that have to be done that day. Then downstairs you go and you're in this frantic push- push mode to get through everything. You push your kids to get ready, push them to get out the door, push yourself to make breakfast, push your husband/partner to do whatever he or she needs to do in the morning, and when all that is done, you jump into the car. In route, you drive through and pick up your $4 cup of coffee, which yet again stimulates the adrenal glands with caffeine. Sitting in traffic you think, "Don't they know I have places to go?" You're completely stressed, and late? You get to the office and to your desk. You sit down and start checking your email, drinking coffee, answering the phone, and setting up a meeting for 2 P.M. this afternoon with your colleague. You look at your desk and there's the huge project—the one you have to get done. The phone rings and it's the plumber. You schedule him for 7 A.M. Saturday morning. You log on and answer more email. Your colleagues come in to chat. When they leave, you look at your project. It is now 12 noon. You have two options: Either go to lunch or go to the gym. You choose to go to the gym. So, you get ready and you go to the gym because you've got to take care of your body. You leave work, get to the gym and start walking on the treadmill. You are thinking: What about the project? What about dinner? You remember Jamie has a birthday party tomorrow! Got to get a present! What about the project? Are we going to do this in April? No, May? No, okay August. Okay, August is a good time for this and you're sweating and you look at your watch, oh-my-gosh it's 12:35 P.M. Okay thirty-five minutes, that's enough time. You're on your way back from the gym and it's time to pick up something to eat because you realize you are starving. You drive through and pick up some fast food on your way back to your desk. You sit down, check your emails, eat your lunch, go to your 2 P.M. meeting that you set-up, talk about the project, come back to your desk, you answer a couple of phone calls, you look at your watch and think, "Oh-my-gosh! It's 3 P.M.! I have to go home, but I'm hungry—did I eat lunch? It's okay if I didn't eat lunch because I didn't work out hard enough." You have to get home because you have to be there to take care of your kids. You rush home, and become super-mom—you make a snack for your children, while thinking about the laundry you have to do, and what you're going to do for dinner, and the project. The kids come home. "Hi kids, how was your day at school? Oh-my-gosh it's Friday. Friday is softball. Let's go to softball. But you have this project to think about. Okay, you'll think about the project at softball." You take the kids to softball. You're at a softball game and your cell phone rings. Oh great! "Hi Debbie, it's so good to talk to you. What do you mean you're redoing the bedroom? Blue carpet? Blue carpet sounds great! Jimmy you got a run!" Meanwhile, you're thinking I can have Marcia help on the project, and we need to pick-up dinner on the way home. "She said what to you? I can't believe she said that! Run, run, go, team, we scored a run!" Okay, August, I'll have Marcia do the project. But what about Jamie's birthday party? Shoot! I need something for that birthday party. We'll do that on the way home. Game's over. "Loved talking to you." You hang up on your friend. You head home. You stop at the grocery store, with kids in tow and get dinner. Once home, you send your kids off. As you're making dinner you're thinking about your project. Your husband comes home. "Hi honey, Sit down and we'll have dinner." Everybody has dinner together. They all get up, the dishes are in the sink, and the laundry is in the washing machine. Now you have a minute to think about the project. "What honey? It's Friday night? You want to go to bed early tonight? Sure, let's go to bed early tonight." You'll think about the project upstairs. So you go upstairs and you get ready for bed. "Oh no! I totally forgot to pick up that present for Jamie. I'll sleep a little late and we'll get it after. Oh shoot, I can't sleep late tomorrow morning—the plumber's coming at 7 A.M.! Why did I do that?" You put on your negligee. You look in the mirror and think, "I think my hips are getting bigger. I have to start spending more time at the gym. My hips are getting so big!" Okay, the project right? You come out of the bathroom saying, "Okay honey, I'm ready for bed."

Question: How are you supposed to be available, present, accessible and enjoy your life when you are never in it? You are just thinking about what comes next. Imagine how people in your life are feeling—trying to get to you when you are buried under all this stuff. They are wondering—*are you under there?*

Paradigm shifting story: Several years ago I had this great boyfriend in New York City. He would come to Newark airport to meet me after a trip, which, if you have ever been to Newark Airport, you know it is a hard place to meet someone. This great boyfriend would always meet me outside the security area.

He would ask, "Hey, honey, how was your trip?"

"It was good, it was fine," I'd reply.

I would come off the plane with my over-the-shoulder travel bag, my handbag on my other shoulder, and my suitcase had been checked.

He would then say, "Let me take that," referring to the heavy over the shoulder travel bag.

I would counter, "No, no I've got it." So I carried it.

We would go downstairs, down the long hallway, and out to the luggage carousel. We would chat a little about the trip and then he would say, "Which bag is yours?"

I would point it out and he'd say, "Let me get it."

My response was always, "No, no, no, I got it."

Sound familiar? And I would reach onto the carousel and grab the bag thinking, "Hey, I have been on the road for four days. I have been carrying this stuff by myself for four days. I do not need your help right now. I can do it myself."

There I am, leaving the airport, with one heavy bag on one shoulder, my handbag on the other shoulder, pulling my suitcase, and struggling out the door.

Fast-forward a few years; I'm coming into Denver International Airport. The new boyfriend meets me outside of security. He asks, "How was your trip?"

I say "Good, thanks."

He says, "Honey that looks heavy, let me carry it for you."

I reply, "Thank you, that would be great. Thank you for helping me." He takes the heavy shoulder bag and we head down to the luggage carousel.

At the luggage carousel, he says, "Which one's yours?"

I point, and he says, "Let me get that."

I say, "Okay." *He* reaches over, *he* pulls the suitcase off the carousel, and *he* is carrying the travel bag on one arm, pulling the suitcase with the other arm, walking next to me and I'm carrying my handbag.

Question: Which woman walking out of the airport is more powerful? I had previously had it all wrong!

Incorrect assumption: Previously I had the idea that the more I did myself—the more I handled alone—the less I asked for help, the more powerful and successful I was. I had assumed, if anybody helped me, the success wasn't mine, and I didn't get to own it.

In the airport scenario, which woman do you want to be—the woman who *allows* the people in her life to help her, or the woman who is dragging her own bags through the airport?

Strategies for living in a feminine paradigm: I am in no way suggesting that women give up any of the advances and rights they have earned and gained. I am suggesting that women can still do everything they do in their lives, but with a slight shift—possibly do it without all of the stress, and struggle and pushing that has cost them so much.

The alarm clock. Most of us have an alarm clock that wakes us up in the morning. If you are one of those people who can wake up by yourself without an alarm, you may want to read on, and see if the methods I suggest below for creating your day might help. When your alarm clock rings it causes adrenaline to flood your body. If your alarm clock makes an annoying sound like "beep beep beep" or any other annoying sound, you will not be relaxed when you wake up.

Strategy: Find an alarm clock that plays the kind of music you like, or one that has a compact disk player that can play soothing nature sounds. Use the snooze button, but not in the way most of us do, where during the amount of time you're snoozing your mind is racing, and you are obsessing with all of the things you have to do.

Instead, after the alarm clock rings, hit the snooze button, take a deep breath, move your fingers, your toes, take another deep breath, and be in your body. As my grandmother used to say, "Every day above ground is a good day." Be in your body for a moment and realize it is a good day. Then use your snooze time to think about all the things you are grateful for. When you do this, what happens *chemically* in your body is the adrenaline subsides and your brain—when you have an attitude of gratitude and happiness—releases seratonin. Seratonin is the chemical that makes you calm, happy, and relaxed. If you spend that snooze time thinking about all the blessings you have in your life, you'll wake up when the alarm rings the next time and your heart will not be racing—you will be calm.

Then, it's time to take your shower. Have you ever taken a shower, and when you get out you can't remember if you washed your hair? Or, have you taken a shower, meant to shave your legs, and when you get out one of them is shaved and the other one is not? When we are in the shower, we are so busy thinking about what we have to do, we are not even "in" the shower. Think about being present in your life. When you are in the shower, you cannot be anywhere else. It's not possible to multi-task. So, while you're in the shower continue that same sense of relaxation and serotonin release. Be in your body. Enjoy the feeling of water. Enjoy the feeling of soap. And if you're a mom with kids and a husband, it may be the only place where they're not going to bother you or ask you for anything. Be *in* it—enjoy.

Next, imagine a morning that began with your being grateful for the people in your life, and now you get to spend time with them. You're still going to get them to do all the things they have to do, but imagine their response to you if you're not in *push, push, push* mode. If you're in gratitude and peace, and you tell everyone what needs to happen, then allow it...imagine their response to you.

I see the woman in her home like the CEO of a company. I believe in the "top down" theory—the energy and attitude of the boss trickles down to the employees. The energy and the attitude of the woman in the house, whether you live alone or you live with others, completely affects everyone in your home.

Traffic: After you get everyone off to work, off to school, and off to where they have to be, you get to go to work. I am still a big fan of coffee so if you want to have your coffee on the way to work, that's fine. Beware; caffeine does affect your adrenal glands, so drink wisely.

If you drive to work in America in the morning between 7 A.M. and 9 A.M. you're going to struggle through traffic. How many of you are surprised every day when there is traffic? Every day there's traffic; and every day you're surprised. This is another time for you to be in your body and choose to be happy. If you are carpooling, hopefully you are with people you like. If you are commuting with people you do not like, do not commute with them anymore. They are causing you excess stress and energy drain.

During your commute, here is what I recommend:

If you are a "book-on-tape" person, get books on tape or compact disk that are educational. If you are a soft music radio listener, listen to soft music. If you are a country music fan, great—listen to whatever relaxes and calms you; you can even try karaoke, which can be fun.

Women naturally create community. The people sitting next to you in traffic can be your community. Have you ever looked at people in traffic? They are so funny—most of them are growling and scowling and complaining on their cell phones. *It's traffic*—it's going to be there. If you're in this great, relaxed space after the morning you just had, look at the person next to you and just smile at them. Give them a little wave. They are going to think you are crazy. Have fun with it! One of my favorite phrases is, "It is none of my business what you think of me." So have fun and create community on your way to work.

Work: If you wake up every morning thinking about going to work and it makes you sick to your stomach, you start sweating, you get a headache and think, "I can't get out of bed—I can't go." I want you to consider doing something else. This is your life—it's your movie, remember? Work is where most of us spend our most concentrated amount of time per week. If it is making you ill to be there, get out.

Men do so well at work because they are single-focused. Men will pick forty-five to sixty minutes to concentrate. Studies show that the human brain can concentrate on one idea or one project for forty-five to sixty minutes.

Strategy: Find a forty-five to sixty-minute block of time for a project. Find a "Do Not Disturb" sign and put it on the outside of your door. If you are in a cubicle and you need to focus, train your colleagues and your friends that when they see your signal—a big red ribbon or a man's tie, *anything* on the edge of your space—to not bother you until it comes down. Give yourself the forty-five to sixty minutes. If you spend an hour in the morning and the same time in the afternoon working on a project, you will not have to take it home. As much as possible, when you are at work, *be at work*. When you are at home, well, you get the idea.

"I need your help": These are four of the most powerful words I know. So many women are afraid to ask for help at work because they fear they will not look as smart, will not look as competent, and will not look as capable as they truly are.

The other side: How do you feel when somebody asks you for help when it's genuinely needed? You're flattered because that person thinks you are smart, knows how good you are, and wants your help. When you ask someone else for help, you give that same gift. So ask your colleagues to help you. If they are better at something than you are, ask them to do it with you, for you, or take on that part of the project because then, everybody wins and looks better. It will not make you look weak. Men do it all the time—they have no issue with it. Ask for help at work, it's really great!

Your health and body: Your body is the transportation for your mind and spirit. It gets you to and from work, home to your partner, to your kids, to play tennis, and whatever it is you are passionate about. You only get one body. Feed it, water it, move it and take care of yourself. There are many resources to get health information. Do what you need to do to take care of your body.

If you find that you're getting really tired in the middle of the day, you may be dehydrated; drink a glass of water. Or it's possible you are protein depleted; a lot of women don't eat enough protein. Eat something high in protein to keep your energy up throughout the day.

Girlfriends: Your friends are in your life to make your life better. Most of us keep our friends, or try to keep our friends forever. Something I read years ago changed that for me, "Everybody is in your life for a reason, a season, or a lifetime." If a friendship has run its course, be clear as to what you want the friendship to look like going forward. Verbalize it and let your friend choose to play in your movie or not. Also, a litmus test for a friendship is: After spending time with her/him, ask yourself, "Do I feel better about myself now or worse?" Notice how you feel each time you leave someone's company. If you are consistently feeling badly about yourself after being with them it may be time to let them go.

Family: Many books have been written on how to make your relationships with your family members work. Let me offer a few tried and true strategies (generously contributed by my friends) for being with your kids:

1. Pick one night a week and have game night—everyone stays home and plays games. You will be with your family in a structured, non-pressured way. You can start with puzzles when the kids are little and move onto Scrabble and Monopoly.

2. Find one thing you have to do at night whether it is the dishes, laundry, or the kid's homework. Pick one child to do that activity with you. Not only

does it teach him or her how to do the dishes and how to do laundry, but you will also have time to be alone with your child. I once heard, "Nothing is more important than stories from a seven-year-old. Whether or not you listen to the story from that seven-year-old, you'll create a different seven-year-old tomorrow."

Intimacy: Men are here because they want to provide for you, they want to protect you, and they want to make you happy. That makes them smile. If they are accomplishing that, and they become your hero for it; if they are making you happy, and you are allowing them to provide for you and protect you, then that is fulfilling both their needs and yours.

If they have chosen you to be their favorite person and their co-star—the person they most want to have dinner with—then acknowledge that they have chosen you and enjoy it. Allow them to make you happy because it gives you freedom to not carry your own bags and to walk out of the airport like a lady with grace.

Exercise: Choose one of the following qualities of femininity and make it your character's motivating force for the day. You'll be amazed at how at ease you will feel. People around you will pick up on that vibration and they will feel comfortable as you are expressing a new facet of who you really are. Try it, it works and can be fun.

Qualities of femininity

Vulnerability: Willingness to expose your true self and true feelings regardless of an imagined risk.

Compassion: Be sympathetic and patient with others' distress with a desire to alleviate it..

Generosity: Be open, giving and sharing. This is accomplished by knowing you have enough for yourself first.

Serenity: Exude calm, peace, and clarity no matter what comes your way.

Allowing/Receiving: Create space in your life for others to do for you and be there for you. Be gracious and accept.

It's a Wrap!

Since you are the director, the producer, the star, the writer, and the casting agent for your own movie, create it exactly how you want it to be. Your movie can bring you experiences, adventures and relationships that help you develop and grow. All this is building toward an ending you will be proud to leave the world with.

And the Oscar goes to.....YOU!

About The Author

Carolyn Strauss

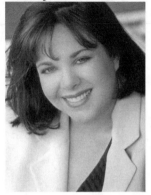

Defying society's narrow, idealized perception of beauty, Carolyn Strauss not only enjoyed a highly successful 20-year career as a plus-size fashion model with the Ford Modeling Agency in NYC, she parlayed that success into The Carolyn Strauss Collection, a multimillion dollar apparel company that is regularly featured on the Home Shopping Network. Her face and voice are familiar to millions of Americans, having appeared on CNN, *Entertainment Tonight, Maury, Sally Jesse Raphael,* and is a frequent guest on many local talk shows. In addition to being the CEO and spokesperson for her company, Carolyn is also an internationally recognized fashion consultant and commentator, certified personal trainer, keynote speaker, and author. Carolyn is a powerfully compelling, effervescent, and entertaining speaker whose entrepreneurial story and original ideas about change and freedom inspire people to change their perceptions of themselves and their relationships to the world. Her uplifting and motivational messages of empowerment, self-acceptance, and personal clarity transform people's lives. Carolyn's background includes a BFA in Theatre from Emerson University; study at the renowned American Academy of Dramatic Arts in New York City; and performances with Chicago City Limits, New York City's longest-running comedy revue. Having made the choice to leave New York City, Carolyn currently lives in Denver, CO.

Carolyn Strauss, President
It's Your Movie™
Denver, CO
Phone: 212.840.1844
Fax: 303.691.6516
CStrauss@CarolynStrauss.com
www.CarolynStrauss.com

Chapter 9

Healthy Thinking Habits:
Seven Attitude Skills Simplified

Cathy Burnham Martin

"Eagles come in all shapes and sizes, but you will recognize them chiefly by their attitudes."
> —Charles Prestwich Scott (1846–1932) British journalist, editor, and politician

"You can make your bed with a smile, or you can make your bed with a frown, but you're going to make your bed." Those are words I heard often from my all-time Great American Mother, Glenna Burnham. She had her hands full with my crummy childhood attitude; but a mere child was no match for this strong, determined woman! Sure, she insisted on having a clean house, but she wanted happy, healthy children even more. My parents' multitude of lessons once learned would make me a far happier, healthier, and more resilient adult.

Medical experts agree that having a positive attitude means getting sick less often and, if sick, being able to recover quickly. Great attitudes are not easy to come by. What's even more annoying is the simple fact that we can't blame a bad attitude on genetics. We can't control what happens to us or around us, but we have complete control over how we respond to it. That response can have an amazing impact on our health, both immediately and collectively.

Think about people with the uncanny ability to roll with the punches. Challenges seem to roll off their backs like water off a duck. However, paddling like crazy underneath the water's surface could result in stomachs twisted into knots or increased risk of heart disease because of inner stress.

When impersonating Fernando Lamas, comedian Billy Crystal said, *"It's better to look good than to feel good, and you look mahhhvelous."* But that was comedy—this is real life. We need to feel good in order to look good, and it all starts with how we think. Healthy eating habits get plenty of attention. Healthy thinking habits should too—that means attitude.

We often hear that success is determined much more by attitude than aptitude or skill. Even noted genius Albert Einstein said, *"Imagination is more important than information."* I call that a ringing endorsement of the idea that attitude beats aptitude.

Generating a great attitude is no small task; it's an ongoing process for the rest of our happy lives. Our human tendency is to resist things that are good for us, which reflects what I call that stubborn sassy streak of youth. As children we were taught *not* to sass, but as American writer, journalist, and humorist Samuel Clemens (known as Mark Twain, 1835–1910) said, *"You should never "sass" old people unless they 'sass' you first."*

The rules have changed—my kind of sass is not only okay, but it's a positively essential part of healthy living. SASS is simply my acronym for Seven Attitude Skills Simplified. Those seven skills are: emPowerment, Planning, Perspective, Positive actions, Persistency, Poise, and Passion. You could call them the "P" vitamins. A minimum daily "P" vitamin requirement hasn't been established, but a healthy and happy, quality life most certainly needs all seven. Their benefits are cumulative, but daily supplements of each are beneficial.

SASS #1—emPowerment

"Only I can change my life. No one can do it for me."

—Carol Burnett (1933–), American actress and comedienne

People often look outside themselves for happiness, for empowerment, for someone to make sense of all the nonsense. Yet, you have complete control over your attitude. Your good or bad attitude is *someone's* decision—make it *yours*.

Why do people feel so powerless? It's been said that if you think you are too small to be effective, you have never been in the dark with a mosquito. Throughout the ages many great minds have commented on our ability to choose how we feel about life and who we are. Below are some cogent statements:

- Ancient Roman philosopher, statesman and humorist Senaca (3 B.C.–A.D. 65)—"*A man is as unhappy as he has convinced himself he is.*"
- U.S. First Lady, human rights activist and diplomat Eleanor Roosevelt (1884–1962)—"*No one can make you feel inferior without your consent. Never give it to them.*"
- Mark Twain—"*The worst loneliness is not to be comfortable with yourself.*"

Empowering yourself means believing in yourself and being the person you want people to know you are. This does *not* mean being perfect. Making no mistakes is NO blessing. We can *correct* mistakes—that's why pencils have erasers. Remember the adage that "anything worth doing is worth doing poorly, until we can learn to do it well." So, step out boldly.

Another key to boosting personal power is to do what *you* expect of *yourself*, rather than what others may expect of you. We tend to get wrapped up in pleasing other people to the point where we're not able to please anyone. If that sounds familiar, STOP. Let it go. If you really want to be able to treat other people fantastically then you must start with yourself.

When we lose that balance we lose perspective—we get stressed. Remember all the talk about "middle child syndrome?" I lived that angst of overcompensating to try and please everyone. I was sad and felt very alone. I worked crazily to do everything well. Though a classic overachiever, I felt I wasn't doing enough. In reality, I had *no* reason to feel that way, but I'd bought into a very self-destructive philosophy. In truth, no one liked me more or less if I did or did not do a multitude of things.

By my pre-teen years, my father compared me to a clock's pendulum that was out of balance. He said my emotional swings needed moderation if I wanted to find happiness. Very correctly he observed that when I was "up" no one could be higher—I was a delight and full of positive energy. But when I was "down" no one could be lower—I was as miserable an adolescent as anyone could hope to never meet. Dad suggested I think about it and see if life wasn't happier if I could get that personal pendulum to moderate and swing more in the middle.

Then I slumped into guilt, thinking I'd actually disappointed everyone I loved. I'd let people down by working so hard to do things I thought would please them. Downward spirals are fast and furious. They may not be logical, but when you are living them, they *are* reality. What we struggle to realize is they don't have to *stay* reality.

We need to forgive ourselves for being human. We need to think logically to get a better foundation, and we need honest emotion to give us true commitment and warmth. Balance helps us open a window in our self-created dark place and let in some light. Only then have we given ourselves the power to grow and develop. Some people call it reinventing yourself. I call it emPowering yourself. Call it anything you like, just do it.

SASS #2—Planning

"Before everything else, getting ready is the secret of success."

—Henry Ford (1863–1947), Founder of Ford Motor Company

Until it's a habit, planning is often easier said than done. The point, however, is undeniable—Plan—Set goals. Determine specific steps needed to reach your goals. Realize that setbacks along the way are natural.

It seems realistic that we don't plan to fail. Failure is usually because we failed to plan. But planning is a learned skill. Many of us never quite master day-to-day time management, never mind long-term goal setting. The key is taking charge of that daily "Must Do list."

I know people who never write down appointments. They don't carry a calendar, and why should they? They'd never look at it anyway. Then they get anxious when they suddenly realize they're late for a commitment or have missed something altogether. They feel frustrated and exhausted much of the time. That's unfortunate, since it's totally avoidable.

There are many things we *can't* control in our lives. Why miss out on something simple that *gives* us control? Maintaining a daily, weekly, monthly, and annual calendar lets us plan ahead, keep buffer time between events, block out personal time, and make family commitments. We keep control and relieve the pressure of panic and rushing.

When we follow a schedule we can make adjustments that work *for* us. We can actually fit more into a day and end up accomplishing much more.

Entrepreneur Dexter Yeager always said, *"True dreams are goals with dates. The rest are just wishes."* So, a little planning can go a long way:

- Write down big and small goals.
- Identify small steps required to accomplish each goal.
- Do the needed tasks to follow the identified steps.
- Set deadlines for yourself. Even jazz pianist and composer Duke Ellington (1899–1974) said, *"I don't need time. What I need is a deadline."*
- Put needed action items in your calendar with blocked out time for each.
- Prioritize your short- and long-term, daily, and lifetime goals.
- Be very specific. "I will try twelve new restaurants within the next twelve months" is better than "I want to find some new places to eat."
- If visual reminders help you stay focused, cut out representative photos or encouraging words and pin them where you'll see them.
- Consider where and when you are most apt to get off track and build up defenses *now* to be ready to fight back *then*.
- Be sure your goals are truly *yours* and not someone else's goals for you.
- Be realistic. Don't overwhelm yourself. The best way to eat an elephant is one bite at a time.
- When you stumble, get back up and start trying again.
- Believe you will win!

Is goal setting really that important? Yes. Plain and simple. As the founder of "Forbes" business and financial magazine, B. C. Forbes (1897–1954) said, *"If you don't drive your business, you'll be driven out of business."* That applies to life. Those who cannot discipline themselves are destined to be disciplined by others. Control your time or others will control it. We've heard these sayings before because they're true. We must not wait for the right circumstances, or day, or mood. Decide that today is yours and move forward.

We never want to just let life happen to us. We'd only end up feeling out of control. Kahlil Gibran, the twentieth century mystic philosopher said, *"We choose our joys and sorrows long before we experience them."* So, set positive goals and then work to make achieving them your reality.

SASS #3--Perspective

"Whether you think you can or think you can't, you're usually right."

—Henry Ford

Whenever we think we're being objective, we should probably think again. As humans, we tend to hold extremely rigid views and opinions. Our innate stubbornness can actually inspire sadness and doubt. We just "hope" we are right. Nagging doubts chip away at our confidence.

When we learn we've been wrong, we choose our response either openly or subconsciously. Sometimes we rationalize the facts so we can justify what we'd believed so strongly was true. We can refuse to shift our perspective because we just don't want to admit we were wrong or had anything to "learn." We puff up and rant and rave, even though that only reveals our stubborn, ignorant, and intolerant side. In truth, these rationalizations deteriorate our self-respect and step heavily on our chances for a consistently good attitude.

Sometimes we shift to recognize a view that we hadn't previously had room for in our minds. We accept facts and open our perspective. We can do this graciously and "eat a little crow," if need be. Humbling ourselves and accepting we are human enables us to grow and learn comfortably.

Permitting ourselves to be enlightened is very healthy. It relieves frustration, helps us laugh at ourselves, and helps us understand others. Laughing at ourselves is particularly important, because it's too easy to take ourselves too seriously. I really like the perspective from French writer Nicolas Chamfort (1741–

1794), *"Swallow a toad in the morning and you will encounter nothing more disgusting the rest of the day."* Now *there's* some food for thought—very "punny," I know.

Allowing new evidence or thinking to change our perspective also means that in future situations we are more likely to be more open minded... to think more calmly and objectively. This lowers stress levels considerably and thus helps us stay healthier. As American author and philosopher Henry David Thoreau (1817–1862) said, *"It's not what you look at that matters, it's what you see."*

Humility was an unexpected perspective gained early as a television broadcaster. There's no escaping the true strength of the human spirit:

- I reported on the sad path of very ill children with timeless souls and unending love, and I marveled at their faithful courage.
- Behind the iron curtain in Moscow, KGB-hounded people looked into my eyes with the most amazing combination of hope and desperation; I was moved beyond words. I've never before felt so powerless, angry, and fortunate all at the same time.
- When nervous faces stepped through the small, early openings in the Berlin Wall into the little island of freedom called West Berlin, I was humbled into tears immediately by the undeserved hugs I received. I was undeserving, but as an American, I was seen as representative of all that America had done to keep hope alive and secure their chance to be free. Humbling indeed, especially when you think about all the people who died.

We all need good doses of perspective—we grow when we allow people to touch us and open our eyes. Thirty-second U.S. President Franklin D. Roosevelt (1882–1945) understood perspective clearly when he said, *"The only limit to our realization of tomorrow will be our doubts of today."* And his First Lady Eleanor Roosevelt knew how to put perspective into action, *"A stumbling block to the pessimist is a stepping stone to the optimist."* We can't eliminate challenges, but we can learn to see the possibilities rather than the impossibilities and improbabilities. And *that* is a good kind of SASSY.

SASS #4—Positive Actions

"The reason why worry kills more people than work is that more people worry than work."

> —Robert Frost (1874–1963), American poet, winner of four Pulitzer prizes

Having knowledge but not applying it is like begging for unrealized potential. As Will Rogers said, *"Even if you're on the right track, you'll get run over if you just sit there."* That's true, but not just any action will suffice. If you row hard with just one oar in the water, you'll go really fast but only in circles. Activity alone doesn't get the job done nor relieve your stress. You need to take the *right* action. That means actually *doing* what you know you should do. And yet, when we do things in our lives that *don't* generate the desired results, why do we so often continue to do those same things? I like Crystal Cathedral minister Dr. Robert H. Schuller's recognition of this human foible, *"It takes guts to get out of the ruts."*

Theoretical physicist and Nobel Prize-winning scientist Albert Einstein (1879–1955), said, *"The definition of insanity is doing the same thing over and over again and expecting a different result."* It's like Charlie Brown banging his head against the tree thinking it will make the tree grow faster. We all know the joke that we're banging our head against the tree because it feels so good when we stop. What we miss sometimes is the great lesson: Don't do it again. Then we can avoid the pain completely.

As humans, it's our birthright to live and learn. Experience is the best teacher, especially when it's someone *else's* experience. Our human stubborn streak often restricts our ability to accept someone else's advice. The sign is meaningless; we have to prove to ourselves that the paint on the bench really is wet.

Positive action steps:

- Find activities that yield positive results; repeat them.
- Recognize activities that drain personal resources—energy, time, attitude, finances—avoid them.
- Polish skills that support positive activities.
- Practice. Practice. Practice.
- Don't give up if not skillful at first. Long before he was famous, the great French sculptor Auguste Rodin (1840–

1917) recognized, *"Nothing is a waste of time if you use the experience wisely."*

If you are in or desire a position of leadership you also need to recognize you have to accept additional responsibility. People follow based on trust and respect. It would be great if all managers had leadership skills. Sadly, we all know managers who are in those roles due to promotions, not leadership ability. We try to understand those people, but we certainly don't want to emulate them.

In any role in life, we can be happier and healthier if we honestly adopt leadership skills. This means:

- Setting the right example
- Supporting other people's efforts
- Delegating all possible activities
- Trusting other people's talents and intentions
- Following through
- Recognizing and rewarding accomplishments of others
- Not procrastinating
- Respecting other people's time
- Practicing good time management

It's easy to get strapped into a false, self-inflicted straight-jacket of stress with the world on our shoulders. Set yourself free and help others do the same by getting your own act together.

You may think following lists and schedules is too restrictive to your freedom. Remember, you can take a train off its tracks—it's free, but it can't go anywhere. So, set a priority to make a schedule to get and stay on track. Review and update your day's plan each morning. Post reminders wherever you need to until following your schedule becomes a habit. Stay on course. If you have five tasks that must be accomplished, don't let yourself get off track, doing items six to ten tasks. Maintain control of your time. Get the "must do" items done first. This lowers stress and actually provides more time to accomplish additional items on your Must Do list and even your Wish To Do list.

Perhaps most important to your good health, especially if you tend toward Type A personality traits, is to let the day come to an end—walk out the door—don't take work home with you. We all need to refresh and recharge. It will all still be there the next day. Live your life in such a way that there just isn't a chance for burning out. That is self-respect.

Another wonderfully refreshing thing happens when you are taking the right actions. You prove naysayers wrong. There are always those ranting about how things *can't* be done, and they are repeatedly interrupted by people doing them! That is not only fun, but it also makes the discipline and effort of doing the right things even more satisfying and personally rewarding.

Regardless of who you are, there's another specific positive action to include on the Must Do list—play. As children, we did this naturally. As we grew into adulthood, most of us were weaned from playing. That's sad. We need to learn to play again and allow ourselves some regular playtime. It doesn't matter what you love to do—just do it. Have fun—laugh out loud—often. Enjoy this time called "Life."

"We do not stop playing because we grow old. We grow old because we stop playing!"

> —Benjamin Franklin (1706–1790) American printer, journalist, author, philanthropist, diplomat, and inventor

SASS #5--Persistence

"I'm a great believer in luck. The harder I work, the more I have of it."

> —Thomas Jefferson (1743–1826) third U.S. President and crafter of the Declaration of Independence

The truth of persistence is that it works and gets the job done. We only get flustered when we stop short of a goal. We plan and prepare for a particular project that's a three-hour task. But, if it turns out to be a five-hour task, we can't win if we give up after four hours. The adage is true that says, *"A big shot is just a little shot that kept on shooting."* Movie fans of the *Star Wars* film "The Empire Strikes Back" remember Yoda's sage remark, *"Do or do not. There is no try."*

So much has been said about being persistent and consistent. In all walks of life they are seen as keys to success, good self-image, and accomplishment. It doesn't matter if we're trying to learn to make a good pasta sauce or master a new computer software program. We discipline ourselves to lose an extra five or ten pounds, but then we return to our old habits and watch every pound return. Why? We failed to develop a positive action plan at which we could be persistent. Honestly, can you think of any skill or endeavor that is not improved by a persistent effort?

Hollywood movie mogul Cecil B. DeMille (1861–1959) said, *"The person who makes a success of living is the one who sees his goal steadily and aims for it unswervingly. That is dedication."*

American self-help author and motivator Zig Ziglar (1926–) noted, *"Others can stop you temporarily—YOU are the only one who can do it permanently."*

And no matter how great a champion you are, the need for persistence doesn't waiver. Consider the great American composer and lyricist Irving Berlin's (1888-1989) words, *"The toughest thing about success is that you've got to keep on being a success."*

The awareness of persistence as a major key has been clear for centuries. American basketball coach Pat Riley (1945–) recognized persistence with his creed, *"Excellence is the gradual result of always striving to do better."* Such thinking is hardly a new concept, since Greek philosopher Aristotle (384 B.C.–322 B.C.) wrote, *"We are what we repeatedly do. Excellence, therefore, is not an act but a habit."* Simplicity comes from having a goal that's important enough to you that you'll persist in the effort needed.

How will this make you healthier? A stagnant pool of water has no sparkle. We are brightest when we are moving toward something that matters to us. Making an effort once, even if successful, is good but less fulfilling than working steadily to improve.

My mother didn't bake the best pies in town on her first attempt. In fact, when she married my father she couldn't cook at all, never mind bake. He taught her the basics, and the rest is history. Her pies became the consistently closest thing to perfection imaginable. I never expect to find a crust that's lighter, flakier, or more delicious than Mom's. Nor am I apt to ever taste fillings that are any fresher, juicier, or so carefully spiced to accentuate natural flavors. She became the undisputed "Best Cook in Town" through persistence.

When I hear someone moaning and groaning about their lack of talent or luck or skill, I know better. They just haven't tried hard enough or long enough. Think of a tennis match. The pros will launch these rocket-propelled ace serves right past their opponents. Do they do this every time? No, but consistent, ace quality serves are surely their goal. They practice their serve hundreds of times each week. They aren't trying to best the 99.9 percent of the population they could beat without practice—they are persistent so they can compete successfully with other professionals. The best want to beat the best, fair and square, with hard-earned skills.

There is great fulfillment and satisfaction for all of us in having persistence pay off with consistent quality. Someone can easily have better raw talent than you do in some area. However, you can zoom past them if you are persistent in the necessary work to improve, and they allow their skills to stagnate. The simple truth is based on simple facts—we succeed when we are willing to do what it takes over and over again.

SASS #6–Poise

"Somehow I can't believe there are many heights that can't be scaled by a man who knows the secret of making dreams come true. This special secret can be summarized in four C's. They are: curiosity, confidence, courage, and constancy, and the greatest of these is confidence."

> —Walt Disney (1901–1966) entrepreneur, animator, and film producer

Poise is a very multi-faceted skill, and it definitely shines from the inside out. When someone is particularly poised, they exude confidence. Poise is never pompous—it is classy. Someone who is poised has magnetism, pizzazz, and chutzpah. A poised person truly lives what I call "The Ten Confidence Commandments:"

1. Physical—Maintain a physical posture and clean presentation to exude a magnetic aura and positive air. As I've often heard said, *"When it comes to staying young, a mind-lift beats a face-lift any day."*
2. Initiative—If you want a competitive advantage in life, demonstrate the foresight of initiative. Numerous writers and leaders hold to variations of the quote, *"Men who try to do something and fail are far better than those who try to do nothing and succeed."*
3. Character—Be of strong character that is built on integrity, trustworthiness and selflessness. Squelch

sarcasm, cockiness and all airs of superiority. In the words of Ralph Waldo Emerson, *"What lies behind us and what lies before us are tiny matters compared to what lies within us."*

4. Knowledge—Keep knowledge as your foundation, preparing well and honing skills; never accept ignorance in yourself, but tolerate it in others. Third Century biographer of Greek philosophers Diogenes Laertius wrote, *"Confidence, like art, never comes from having all the answers; it comes from being open to all the questions."*

5. Commitment—Give whatever it takes. With full commitment you can live well with yourself, regardless of the results. In the words of Italian Renaissance architect, inventor, sculptor, and painter Leonardo da Vinci (1452–1519), *"Obstacles cannot crush me. Every obstacle yields to stern resolve. He who is fixed to a star does not change his mind."*

6. Steadiness—Keep cool under pressure. During the birth of the United States, American writer and philosopher Thomas Paine (1737–1809) said, *"I love men who can smile in trouble, who can gather strength from distress, and grow brave by reflection."*

7. Teamwork—Be a cooperative believer in teamwork, surrounding yourself with positive people and choosing supportive friends. NFL football coach George H. Allen (1922–1990) said, *"Football isn't necessarily won by the best players. It's won by the team with the best attitude."*

8. Expectation—Live with great expectation and positive anticipation of what you want; claim the positive. In his book *Seeds of Greatness,* motivational expert Denis Waitley wrote, *"Life is a self-fulfilling prophecy: You won't necessarily get what you want in life, but in the long run, you will usually get what you expect."*

9. Perseverance—Discipline yourself to persevere to overcome all struggles and challenges. British author, journalist, politician, Nobel Prize winner and Prime Minister Sir Winston Churchill (1874–1965) said, *"Courage is going from failure to failure without losing enthusiasm."*

10. Sportsmanship—Become a "Morale Booster Extraordinaire" by lifting others up and celebrating their successes. Consider the words of American novelist Edith Wharton (1862–1937), *"There are two ways of spreading light: to be the candle or the mirror that reflects it."*

When we have true confidence, we possess that elusive quality called poise. Because the skills that build confidence from the inside out are all learnable, anyone can have this poise. The more poised a person is, the healthier they tend to be also.

SASS #7--Passion

"There is no greatness without a passion to be great."

—Anthony Robbins, motivational speaker

The premise of passion in success has been bantered about and debated for generations. Logic devotees tend to resist the thought of enthusiasm or anything emotional having a positive influence. For me, the enthusiasm of passion is the simplest key to attitude beating aptitude. Consider Candidate A versus Candidate B:

Candidate A	Candidate B
Basic skills and little experience	Top skills and great experience
Sparkle in the eyes	Distrust in the eyes
High energy	Slouches; appears unsure
Positive conversation	Naysayer
Bright and genuine smile	Terse, all-business expression
Seeks and sees the good in situations	Thinks positive thinkers are pushovers
Wonderful sense of humor	Polite laughter at best
Accepts change as growth potential	Resists change as a threat
Even and upbeat mood	Brooding and changeable moods
Thoughtful	Generates tension in others
Makes people feel relaxed	Guarded and careful
Open and honest	Walks on people
Lifts other people up	

It's your choice. It doesn't matter whether you're considering a politician, friend, co-worker, committee member, employee, or boss, Candidate A is far more enthusiastic than Candidate B. Candidate A can be trained for the skills and can gain the experience. Though Candidate B has skills, it's pretty tough to train for attitude. Which one would you want on your team?

Both enthusiasm and misery are extremely contagious. The choice is yours as to how you will infect your world. In truth, some rather powerfully successful people and logical thinkers have *insisted* on enthusiasm:

- Henry Ford—*"You can do anything if you have enthusiasm. Enthusiasts are fighters, they have fortitude, they have staying qualities. Enthusiasm is at the bottom of all progress! With it, there is accomplishment. Without it there are only alibis."*
- American football coach Vince Lombardi (1913–1970)—*"If you aren't fired with enthusiasm, you will be fired with enthusiasm."*
- Business tycoon Malcolm Forbes—*"Men who never get carried away should be."*
- Albert Einstein—*"There are only two ways to live your life. One is as though nothing is a miracle. The other is as though everything is a miracle."*

Life is truly a matter of how we choose to look at it. The same negative circumstances can be applied to two different people with dramatically different results. Why? Because we have free will—we can each choose how we react—we can tremble and stay a victim, we can lash out with defiance, or we can learn new strengths and wisdom and move on.

For some perspective on looking at life with passion, consider:

- Helen Keller (1880–1968), deaf-blind American author, activist and lecturer—*"Life is either a daring adventure, or nothing."*
- Mario Andretti (1940–), American racing driver—*"If everything's under control, you're going too slow."*
- Mark Twain—*"It's not the size of the dog in the fight, it's the size of the fight in the dog."*
- Robert F. Kennedy, (1925–1968) US Attorney General—*"Only those who dare to fail greatly can ever achieve greatly."*

- Billie Jean King, (1943–) American tennis champion—*"Be bold. If you're going to make an error, make a doozy, and don't be afraid to hit the ball."*
- Walt Disney—*"It's kind of fun to do the impossible."*

A happy, healthy life is not the result of meek thinking. Live boldly. Thirty-sixth U.S. President Lyndon Johnson said, *"I'd rather give my life than be afraid to give it."* That rings of patriotism. *My* version of the quote reflects the need to live with passion. I like to say, *"I'd rather live my life than be afraid to live it."*

To the spirit of adventure in our passion for living we should also add a large helping of humor. No other single tool is more valuable in our quest to live well. People who scowl aren't able to enjoy the healing power of humor. It reflects the old saying, *"Growl all day and you'll feel dog-tired all night."* It's a simple fact that an upbeat attitude helps make light work of any task.

Our health benefits greatly when we add laughter to our lives. That's why a good comedian is so refreshing. Day-to-day living can be highly stressful. Just watch news on television and you'll see our human dark side at work. Life's miseries are displayed boldly and repeatedly, because bad news draws us in. Our attitude and health both suffer if we forget that it's just another program fighting for a share of splintering viewer numbers. Though you won't typically see it on television, the vast majority of real life is filled with positive events, people helping people, community successes, kids who are *not* stealing cars or overdosing on drugs, politicians who are *not* cheating or stealing, schools that are safe and productive, companies that are honest, and volunteers who enthusiastically work to boost other people's quality of life.

Four-time Best Actress Oscar-winner Katharine Hepburn (1907–2003) advised, *"Life can be wildly tragic at times, and I've had my share. But whatever happens to you, you have to keep a slightly comic attitude. In the final analysis, you have got not to forget to laugh."* Or, as American comedian Flip Wilson (1933–1998) put it, *"Funny is an attitude."* We need to exercise our attitudes just as we should exercise our bodies. Or, as editor Norman Cousins (1915–1990) put it, *"Laughter is inner jogging."* It's all a matter of choice. In the same way that we choose to be a good or bad role model, we choose to have a good or bad attitude. Choosing positive passion boosts our success, happiness, and health immeasurably.

In SASS Number One, I told you about my father's clock pendulum example as he tried to teach me moderation. Because I was a brat, I stubbornly defied what I recognized as good advice. But because it made sense to me, I quietly worked on creating a moderate swing in the *upper*, more positive mood area. Sure enough, I gradually learned how to be a happier person *every* day. Now, this was not an overnight transformation by any means, but it worked. Decades later I still moderate in that upper range. If I'm having a bad day, my husband says I have to tell him. And my bad days only last for a couple of hours.

There came a day in the mid-1980s when I read an article in *USA Today* that noted, *"Less than two percent of Americans wake up happy."* I was truly taken aback. I knew I was different, but I hadn't realized just *how* different. I don't need a cup of coffee to get in step with the morning; I wake up ready to roll. Better health? Absolutely. Higher resiliency? Unquestionably. Try it; you'll like it.

There's another exciting benefit to the power and purpose that positive passion brings to life—youthful vitality. Though I'm in my fifties at the time of this writing, people are surprised whenever they learn my age. I've always presumed that I've looked my age at every age. Both friends and strangers correct me regularly. This is not attributable to a great diet or stress-free living, I can assure you. My firm belief is that the big difference is a great attitude—a true passion for living.

If I'm having a "down" time, I not only feel slow and low, but the mirror reflects a face that looks twenty years older! I see my sallow complexion, no sparkle or vitality in my eyes, an expressionless mouth. Yuck! Who is *that*?! What I realize is that my exterior is reflecting what's inside. My enthusiasm is low, and it shows. This is true for all of us.

Enthusiasm to me *is* passion. People with positive passion for life do appear and feel more vigorous and more healthy—at every age. I sum up the simplicity of the skill of passion with the words commonly attributed to Watterson Lowe, *"Years may wrinkle the face, but to give up enthusiasm wrinkles the soul."*

With the Seven Attitude Skills Simplified, you're on your way to reducing stress and loading your life with control, quality, and enthusiasm. These "P" vitamins definitely keep our attitudes healthy too. Put a little SASS in *your* life and enjoy a healthier you.

About The Author

Cathy Burnham Martin

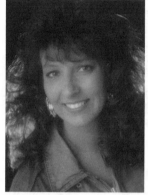

Cathy Burnham Martin has long been dubbed "The Morale Booster" for her outstanding work as a business communicator, motivator, and senior executive speech and media coach. A television broadcaster since the early 1980s, she founded SpeakEasy Communications Management in 1994 to foster stronger public speaking and broadcast media skills in the corporate environment. She also has taught persuasive speaking and com- munication on college campuses. As co- author of *The Communication Coach* in 1998, her tips on "Taming the Media Monster" were highlighted. Cathy has also written dozens of award-winning documentaries, TV specials, and episodes for television focusing on people, events that positively changed lives, culture, fact, fiction, and folklore. A high-energy, high-impact speaker, Cathy has been a professional member of the National Speakers Association since 1995, drawing strong testimonials from her informative and entertaining key- notes and workshops. Popular topics include "Recruit – Retain – Revitalize," "Twisting Like a Pretzel Without Losing Your Salt," "Pur- pose, Power and Passion," and "Growing GREAT Leaders."

Cathy Burnham Martin
SpeakEasy Communications Management
Wellington Trade Center
27 Lowell Street, Suite 201
Manchester, NH 03101
Phone: 888.569.1212
Fax: 888.568.1212
Email: speakeasy123@aol.com
www.speakeasy123.com

Chapter 10

Bio Cranial Therapy for a Pain-Free, Healthy Life

Dr. Stuart Marmorstein

I remember it as though it were yesterday, even though it has been about seven years since I first floated above Dr. Robert Boyd's treatment table after he worked on me. At least, that's what it felt like when I received my first "Bio Cranial correction." It was as though he had given me a sacred initiation into areas of my physicality that had previously been off limits to me. It felt as though I had finally been awarded a rich inheritance that had always rightfully been mine, an inheritance someone or something had unfairly held just out of my reach. I experienced a sense of physical, mental, emotional, and spiritual ease. The ache I was sometimes accustomed to in my lower back completely vanished. My jaw glided open and closed with a remarkable smoothness despite a serious injury that had left it painful for years. My neck turned freely in all directions. And my vision was clearer—in more ways than one.

This all transpired in less than three minutes! There were no popping or cracking sounds and at no time did Dr. Boyd make contact with my jaw, back or neck. What he did felt like a simple and fairly firm stretch. All of the work was focused on my cranial (head) bones. At that time, I had already been a practicing chiropractor for about twenty years. I had already taught postgraduate seminars for chiropractors (including cranial work) and had mingled with and traded treatments with many of the "hotshots" from the chiropractic and bodywork lecture circuits. None of these other treatments had changed my body in any significant way for any meaningful length of time. Since Dr. Boyd's first treatment, my sense of well-being has only increased. It was the perfect time in my life for such a teacher to appear for me.

Dr. Boyd, an osteopath from the United Kingdom of Great Britain (U.K.) has pioneered a natural therapeutic approach for bringing about radical healing changes in the body. It is "radical" in the original sense of the word that means, "getting to the root of the problem." If you want to get rid of the weeds growing in your garden, you don't snip off the top of the weed—you dig up the root. Dr. Boyd's Bio Cranial System (BCS) brings new hope to people who have been everywhere and done everything to help themselves, but to no avail. This approach is also bringing new hope to the doctors who never stopped caring, but who always wondered why their clinical results were often temporary at best.

As I pursued my own re-educational journey with Dr. Boyd, I learned his BCS went far beyond helping banged-up baby boomers like me. Its scope is breathtaking! First of all, it does help pain by getting right to its source. We're talking about every type of pain: fibromyalgia (FM), with its pain all over the back, neck, shoulders, buttocks and legs (and the fatigue that goes with it); trigeminal (trifacial) neuralgia bad enough to make the light touch of bedclothes feel like a lightning bolt; sciatic pain throbbing in the leg; blinding migraines that would make the desperate act of suicide look like a viable option to consider; and post-surgical pain that wasn't supposed to be there any more. Bio Cranial treatments have been able to completely and permanently relieve these various kinds of pain.

The BCS would be miraculous enough if it were merely the greatest natural pain reliever mankind has ever seen; but diabetes, eczema, menstrual and menopausal problems, heart and breathing problems, hiatus hernia and acid reflux "disease"? Come on—how could that be? Well, it *is*. Archimedes, who lived from 287 B.C. to 212 B.C., was a great scientist and inventor. He is quoted as saying, "Give me a lever long enough and a fulcrum on which to place it, and I shall move the world." Robert Boyd, D.O., found the lever and fulcrum to roll away the boulder from the cave where our health has been imprisoned. After several Bio Cranial corrections, all we have to do is walk through that opening into the light and reclaim the abundant life that is our birthright and inheritance.

A Last, A Not-So-Nostalgic Look at Where We've Come From: Is This What You Call Health Care?

We "Baby Boomers" like to feel good and stay active. Unfortunately, people of all ages—including baby boomers—have become far too casual about taking medications to "solve" all of our problems. We do not need to look very far to find drugs. Megadrugstores seem to spring up on every vacant piece of land in America. The big chain grocery stores have their own pharmacy sections, as do the Wal-Mart stores and their competitors. Is it too difficult to find what we're looking for in our own backyard—drugs are on sale just over our borders in Canada and Mexico; they are also readily available through the Internet.

Oh, to feel good again! Which formula should we take for our back pain, heartburn, migraine headaches, anxiety, depression, cramps, or our inability to sleep, lose weight or maintain intimate relations? What did the television say I should ask my doctor for, and what side effects will it give me? I can't remember: perhaps my amnesia is a side effect? The microscopic print on the packaging and the television announcer who is talking so fast he sounds like a tobacco auctioneer both say I could develop dry mouth, headache, itchiness, kidney failure, or have a stroke. I should use extra caution if I'm pregnant, lactating, if I sleep between three and twelve hours per night or if I weigh between fifty and 300 pounds. Never mind, I don't even have the energy to go up and down the aisles of Drug Depot looking for it—they should have a Starbucks in this place!

Welcome to medicine in the twenty-first century with its gleaming hospital towers full of high tech equipment and highly trained sub-sub-specialists and all their support personnel. They can scan or scope every cubic centimeter of our bodies, and can sift through our fluid and tissue samples for the answer to the all-important question: What's wrong with me? Sometimes, when they are done searching, they will have found a real crisis to handle and will do so skillfully and admirably. We should all be grateful for their work and dedication. Sometimes, however, we are only left with a complicated-sounding name for our condition; and little insight into its origin, how to handle it without throwing the body into further imbalance, or how to prevent it.

If our modern approach to health care is succeeding, then why are we putting so many of our school children on Ritalin? Is some new strain of virus to blame for hyperactivity and learning disabilities? Why is scoliosis so prevalent in young spines? Why are there so many new cases of diabetes and asthma in people of all ages? Why do the statistics indicate that so many of us are overweight and depressed? Have you lost loved ones to heart disease or cancer? Do you find it disheartening that in such a prosperous country as ours, we have failed so miserably to regain our health and to maintain it? And can we afford to have ever-increasing portions of our population on disability or in long-term care facilities?

A Refreshingly Brilliant Answer: It *is* All in Your Head.

Treasure hunting is not for the faint of heart or intellect—especially when the treasure contains the power to unlock our healing potential at a level the human race has never known.

Dr. Robert Boyd, an osteopath from the Emerald Isle, knew in his heart and mind that this hidden treasure was real. He knew that once he found it, he could profoundly change people's lives. He perseveres in his search despite many seemingly insurmountable obstacles. Finally, this humble doctor found the treasure that was hidden in plain sight. By seeing and understanding the ordinary human head in an extraordinary way, Dr. Boyd discovered an amazing way to help suffering people feel and function normally again, even after a lifetime of pain and poor health.

When people heard about the country doctor who helped patients with all manner of woes by working on the bones of the head, they might have found the notion odd at first. Real results, however, lead to big reputation, and Dr. Boyd started getting one. Soon patients were arriving at his clinic from around the globe with problems that other doctors had failed to help. Their ailments ran the gamut from knee pains to eczema, from sciatica to diabetes, from anxiety to facial pain, from learning disabilities to frozen shoulders to incontinence, menstrual pain, migraines, and ulcers. The list of conditions he had success with was endless. The unusual thing about his method was that no matter what problem the patient presented, he would listen carefully and then go to work on his patient's head! The knee pains and the eczema got better. The patients felt better than they had in years. Wisely, Dr. Boyd never made any claims of cures or took any credit for all of the healing taking place—he just quietly did his work, which he termed "Bio Cranial Therapy." His practice thrived and life was both good and busy.

One day, Dr. Boyd had a thought that disturbed his peace of mind: What would happen to this treasure he had found were he to be hit by the proverbial bus? He knew he couldn't keep the discovery of a lifetime to himself. How easy it would have been to stay home and let the patients flock to him! The thought certainly tempted him. Could he even communicate his unique and revolutionary concepts and procedures to other doctors? Who would be open-minded enough to take his radical ideas seriously? Could he teach the Bio Cranial System to anyone else? He knew he had to try.

There isn't enough space here to describe the trials and tribulations that Dr. Boyd and Vera, his devoted wife of more than fifty years, have gone through together in order to deliver Bio Cranial Therapy to the world. Through their tireless efforts and sacrifices, this one man's brilliant vision has been transformed into the most exciting natural healing art humanity has ever known. This precious gift has been painstakingly safeguarded for future generations, and a growing nucleus of doctors is making history by reproducing the results Dr. Boyd started having in the U.K. during the last two decades of the twentieth century.

To perpetuate this work, Dr. Boyd has founded The Bio Cranial Institute (BCI), headquartered in Houston, Texas. The BCI now offers training to qualified doctors across several disciplines who are ready to embrace the unfamiliar but startlingly hopeful principles of life and healing that Dr. Boyd has discovered and developed. A handpicked faculty works closely with small groups of doctors in training to ensure they can reproduce the crucial manual skills needed to deliver excellent Bio Cranial Corrections with consistency. Thus far, Dr. Boyd has personally participated in the training of each Certified Bio Cranial Practitioner.

In addition to being a brilliant scientist and innovator, Dr. Boyd is an excellent and patient teacher. Having known and worked with him and Vera for quite a few years, I am happy to report that neither of them ever acquired the ego or arrogance that so often accompanies greatness. This patience with their students is necessary because Bio Cranial procedures are exactingly precise and require a type of intense but relaxed focus during delivery to the patient. Sometimes the students think they are being taught to ride a bicycle—on a tightrope!

The Boyds are among the most pleasant, friendly, and helpful people I've ever met. They have taught their instructors by example how to convey this work and its refreshingly natural philosophy to aspiring doctors so they can leave the training program with skill, grace, and confidence.

These re-educated doctors have gone back to their practices with renewed zeal and have been astonished by how quickly their patients get better—and stay better! In fact, many of the doctors' own personal chronic pains and health challenges have already improved during the course of their training! As we will soon discuss, the Bio Cranial System addresses human structure and function at a much deeper level than we were previously able to access. Speedy results and rapid stabilization are hallmarks of the Bio Cranial System. Our approach is fundamentally different from medicine, acupuncture, chiropractic adjusting, osteopathic manipulation, massage, energetic healing, and even other forms of cranial work you may have encountered.

As we explore how and why the Bio Cranial System works, it will become clear why patients of all ages are choosing this safe, drug-free and non-invasive healing art to get well and stay well; and why you and your family will want to...well...have your heads examined! Whether you have endured recurrent bouts of back trouble, fibromyalgia, or fatigue, or you feel great and want to improve your athletic or academic performance, the Bio Cranial System provides answers.

Jackie Kidder's Story Changes *my* Life

I was one of the early adopters who decided to use the Bio Cranial System in my chiropractic practice. Dr. Boyd exposed me to his theories and taught me how to use his approach to correct cranial imbalances. Through improving the alignment and motion of the skull's interlocking plates, patients got better. In fact, they were getting more profound and rapid results than I had ever seen in a quarter century of practice; and the results tended to last.

One day, Mark Kidder brought his wife, Jackie, to see me as a patient. It is said that when the student is ready, the teacher will appear. This has been a recurrent theme in my own life. My patients have taught me more about the limits of human endurance than I wish to experience personally; and more about the courage of the human spirit to persevere through years of mind numbing struggle with pain and other symptoms. Jackie and Mark have taught me that the tools my mentor, Dr. Boyd, gave me are enough—not just enough for the everyday problems I see as a chiropractor, but for conditions that severely limit a person's capacity to enjoy life here on this earth.

Whenever I reread her story, it is hard to imagine that the vibrant, healthy, fit, and pain-free woman I know now went through these horrors. Warning: Jackie's heroic odyssey is sometimes shocking but, as I was to learn later, not that unusual. The following is an abbreviated version of Jackie's story about overcoming a nine-year $100,000 case of fibromyalgia. For the full version in Mark's words, you can visit www.drstuart.net/jackie.htm.

Mark describes how it all began: "My wife, Jackie, was a very active and physically fit woman who felt great physically and mentally. She loved life! She worked out four to five days a week with hour-long aerobics classes and a weight-training plan. She ate healthy foods, didn't smoke, and took no medication at all. She cut the grass, washed the cars, cooked every night, and kept the house neat as a pin. In short, she was unstoppable!

"On July 23, 1995, while looking for a birthday card in a Wal-Mart store in Katy, Texas, she tilted her head up and 'saw stars.' She was in so much pain, she had to sit on the floor in the store for about fifteen minutes. She left the cards behind and barely made it home. At that moment our lives were instantly changed forever."

Jackie developed "acute, continuous, sharp, shooting, and burning pain in the back of her neck, shoulder blades, and upper back." She also started getting debilitating migraine headaches two to three times per month that would often cause her to throw up uncontrollably because the pain would be so intense. The muscles in her neck, shoulder blade, and upper back areas were in constant spasm, escalating the pain levels. The knots spread into her hamstrings and calves. Soon she had to endure "Restless Leg Syndrome."

Jackie and Mark thought she must have a ruptured disc in her neck pressing on nerves. They had never heard of fibromyalgia, so they sought treatment for a disc problem. However, a neurosurgeon had all of the usual scans performed and pronounced Jackie "neurologically sound." The Kidders were shocked by this and began to visit a series of other doctors. Two neurologists, an endocrinologist, and an internal medicine specialist all told them that Jackie had fibromyalgia (FM). She was given injectable Imitrex for the migraines, Carisoprodol (a powerful muscle relaxer) and Lortab (an addictive pain medication). As the condition worsened, more and more powerful medications were introduced. So far the diagnosis was still fibromyalgia with Myofascial Pain Syndrome.

Jackie consulted a rheumatologist, who said, "No Lupus—a touch of osteoarthritis." He prescribed a TENS Unit (Electrical Stimulation of Muscles) and Celebrex anti-inflammation medication (since taken off the market because of side effects.) Guaifenesin was also prescribed as it purportedly helped FM sufferers. None of this provided any measurable relief. Jackie was referred to one of the top pain management specialists in Houston.

By now, Lortab and other pain medications no longer worked effectively so she was put on a 75µg (seventy-five micrograms) per hour Duragesic (morphine) patch that was normally reserved for cancer patients. The patch barely helped the pain, and she was completely debilitated.

They decided to try chiropractic, and Jackie saw a doctor of chiropractic who treated one of the professional sports teams in Houston three times a week. She got minimal relief, which did not last very long. They tried a world-renowned oriental medicine specialist for acupuncture twice a week. She got some relief that was always gone within one hour of the treatment. Then, there was an osteopath who prescribed "natural hormones" and a very expensive regimen of vitamins, minerals, herbs, etc., which did not help at all.

A Pain Management Physician (specialist) evaluated Jackie's worsening pain level at a level of nine and a half on a scale of ten. Each day Jackie's excruciating pain wore her down a little more. Finally, the doctor decided to take a drastic step. He put her in a hospital for one day a week for three weeks to do the following procedure: He put her under general anesthesia in an operating room, placed her on her stomach, secured her hands behind her back, securely strapped her body and head to the table, threaded a catheter into her cervical spinal column and injected her with the latest and most expensive, cutting edge steroidal concoction at the "point of pain."

Mark explains: "Why tie her down to the table? Because when the catheter is being threaded through her spinal column, there is precious little extra room at that part of the spine (in her neck). If she were to partially awake in a 'twilight conscious' state during the procedure and move her body in any way, the catheter could irreversibly damage her spinal cord. We both signed all types of waivers of liability to protect the doctor and hospital if this happened. This was pretty scary, but what was our option? We happily risked paralysis to get rid of this miserable pain—obviously we were very desperate—it was our only hope at the time. We had to try something!"

"The outcome? Well, after operation number one, she had no pain for the next week. She was pain free after operations numbers two and three so we were very encouraged! However after operation number three her pain returned with the same vengeance as before about ten days after the third and final procedure. The total cost of all three procedures: $30,000. Now she had all of the same pain, but she also had two nice parting gifts—she had quickly gained twenty pounds and she now had patches of dark facial hair appearing. One good thing: at least the $30,000 bought her relief for *ten days—$3,000 per day!*"

"We tried other things: yoga, nutrition, diet, visible light therapy, etc. We tried everything that every quack will sell you for hope. She found no relief and she was still on a morphine patch. She was absolutely miserable."

The horror story continued. Jackie went to a third neurologist, who put her on a different cocktail of medications; and she had to go through withdrawal from morphine. By the summer of 2000 (five years later!) the Kidders had already spent more than $100,000, and all they had to show for it was Jackie's pain was now "tolerable." She was still extremely heavily medicated, and life was limited.

Then in March of 2004, Jackie had a terrible setback. Mark writes, "We immediately went back to neurologist number three. The neurologist increased all her doses of medication by fifty percent and added to 'the drug cocktail' the maximum dose of Neurontin (3600 micrograms per day). Jackie was taking all of this medication and was still really in a lot of pain. She was very afraid that she would be returning to the morphine patch. Her head, neck, and upper back were in constant pain, and her neck, hamstrings, and calves were in knots again. Her ring and middle fingers on her left hand were numb. Her left arm from her hand to her neck hurt so much she could hardly lift it (her arm was so weak that she could not pick up and hold a cup of coffee with her left hand). She was so uncomfortable she could not sleep in bed and slept only a couple of hours each night sitting up in her recliner."

Mark searched the Internet incessantly, looking for possible answers. The FM support groups didn't really offer them much hope. They then found my website and decided to try Bio Cranial Therapy. At this point, what was there to lose?

Something dramatic happened after her first visit: Here is Mark's description: "Now, as a reminder, Jackie was taking eight Lortab (pain) pills per day, tranquilizers, Neurontin, anti-depressants, etc. She took a dose of this cocktail that morning before going for her first Bio Cranial treatment. After the treatment and into the afternoon, she was abnormally quiet and still. She appeared to be a little "out of sorts" and quietly watched television. At about five-thirty she looked at me and said, 'I don't want to jinx this and I'm almost afraid to say it, but I don't have any pain!'

"I damn near fell out of my chair! She was so happy that her pain was 'gone,' she started to cry (and so did I). She told me that even though her next dose of medication was due shortly after lunch she didn't take any of it. It was now five-thirty, she had no pain and now she was afraid to move out of her chair for fear that the pain would come back. She hated to even go to the bathroom for fear of jeopardizing her relief!

"At about seven-thirty, she looked at me and said, 'Hon, I'm so sleepy. I'm going to bed.' To bed—hell! She had not been able to sleep in the bed for eight weeks! (Remember, she was sleeping in her recliner only a couple of hours per night for the past two months). She crawled into bed, rolled over on her *left* shoulder (the one that hurt so much she could hardly touch it), and immediately fell asleep."

Jackie slept for fifteen and a half hours! She said she had not slept that well in years. She described a "soreness" in her neck and upper back, but not much more than that. When Mark asked her what she wanted to do, she wanted to go shopping.

Mark relates, "We had a wonderful 'pain free' weekend. Early the following week, she had a little pain return just like Dr. Marmorstein had predicted (nothing like it was before) and she went in for another treatment. Each week the pain-free periods grew longer and longer, and when the pain returned days later, it was less than the previous week. In about two weeks, feeling came back in her fingers (the neurologist projected that the feeling in her fingers would not return for four to six months). Her migraines immediately stopped after her first Bio Cranial Therapy treatment. She had experienced migraines twice per month over the last nine years and she has not had one migraine in the two months."

I am delighted to report that since Mark wrote this, Jackie now comes to see me every month or two, and has never felt better. She has no pain, takes no medications, and is back to working out regularly, running a business, and having a normal life. They even enjoyed a vacation in Jamaica together. I would also like to point out that Jackie is an excellent patient who takes responsibility for her self-care in other ways, and maintains a good attitude. While Jackie experienced miraculous relief early in her care, she has continued with treatment in order to maximize the benefits she can receive from further opening and unwinding of the cranio-sacral system. Every patient is unique, and his or her healing process will progress at its own rate and in its own time.

The Kidders are wonderful people who have done everything they can to spread the word about the success Jackie has experienced with the Bio Cranial System. Through their efforts information has reached patients with fibromyalgia and other chronic pain syndromes from all over the world. Their story will be published in a scientific journal during the coming year, which will focus the attention of other doctors on the necessity of learning how to apply the Bio Cranial System.

You now know how the lives of Jackie and Mark Kidder have changed, but how has my own life changed through what happened for them? Though I've now treated thousands of other patients with Bio Cranial work, I have a new and deeper respect for the gift of understanding about this extraordinary therapy method Dr. Boyd has given us. My gratitude for this knowledge and for the healing power God has placed inside each one of us has solidified my commitment to see this work become available to everyone in the world who needs and deserves it. Why should people continue to suffer needlessly year after year, when Bio Cranial Therapy can make it possible to restore their health?

While Jackie's story is unusually dramatic, it exemplifies a powerful universal truth: All healing comes from within! Bio Cranial practitioners are leading a natural healing revolution that can change the world, because it is based on unchanging principles.

Understanding The Bio Cranial System

What did Dr. Boyd see that everyone else had missed? Look at your own reflection in a mirror. Study that familiar face you see looking back at you, that you've applied makeup to, or shaved, or washed countless times. If you are like most people, you'll see surface features such as your complexion or a dimple. What Dr. Boyd sees is the bone structure of the face and head. Then beneath that he sees a throbbing, living, pumping universe of membranes, tissues and fluid; all within a head comprised of many bones moving rhythmically together and apart in three dimensions. This strange, secret world that surrounds and protects our brain turns out to be the key player in this story of the Bio Cranial System.

The Quickie Cranial Anatomy Tour

The head of a living human adult weighs between twelve and sixteen pounds. It is actually quite heavy—like a bowling ball. The skull is composed of twenty-two bones (not counting the small bones inside the ears). Contrary to what many people think, these skull plates are not completely fused, even during adulthood. They take part in a slight, rhythmic, involuntary movement, allowing the skull to expand and contract. This movement is vital to all life processes in the body.

A special bone on the back and bottom part of the skull is called the occipital bone, or *"occiput."* There is a unique joint between the occiput and the top bone in the neck that allows our heads to rotate and tilt in many directions. Early anatomists named the top bone in the neck the "Atlas." In Greek mythology, Atlas was one of the Titans. He held the world (sometimes pictured as the earth or as the earth and sky) on his shoulders, as the atlas (or top neck vertebra) holds up our head. When we are out of balance, it can be quite a strain for us to do this!

Inside the skull is the brain, which the Atlas—occiput—protects. The brain floats in a protective cushion of cerebrospinal fluid (CSF), which flows through certain spaces surrounding the brain and spinal cord. The CSF also fills open spaces (ventricles) inside the brain. The largest part of the brain is divided into the left and right cerebral hemispheres, which control most of our thought and sensory processes. Some areas within each hemisphere have been "mapped" and correspond with certain body functions for which they seem to be responsible.

Below them, the brain stem controls such vital functions as breathing and the heartbeat. It anchors the brain to the other part of the central nervous system—the spinal cord—and acts as the main circuit for all brain activity.

Twelve pairs of cranial nerves, emerging from the base of the brain and the brain stem, transmit nerve impulses for vision, hearing, smell, eye movement, and many other important body functions.

The skull also contains the pituitary gland and the hypothalamus which are both instrumental in regulating the hormonal system, temperature, appetite, and other critical control mechanisms.

Nothing in all of creation compares to all of this, and yet this still doesn't explain how a Bio Cranial doctor can use a seemingly simple, but exceedingly precise, physical procedure that can change our total health picture. So, let's look at that.

Imagine you are walking a very large and muscular dog. If you and the dog are relaxing and looking at the ripples on a lake, the leash will hang to the ground, completely slack. If you and the dog are walking together at the same speed in the same direction, the walk will continue to be enjoyable for both of you and the leash will be slack. Suppose you see a friend a short distance away and want to walk over toward them to say hello. Your canine friend, however, has become fascinated by some exotic scent in the grass. He does not want you to go visit with your friend, unless you want to let go of the leash—definitely not an option. The leash becomes tighter and tighter as you and the dog each want to pursue happiness in your own individual way. He is just too strong and heavy to force him to follow you; what do you do? You reach into a little bag containing his favorite doggie treat, and lead him over toward where your friend is waiting for you, and the slackness returns to the leash.

The SECRET Cranial Anatomy Tour: The Reciprocal Tension Membrane System

There is a membrane (rather than a dog leash in the example above) attached to the inside of the cranium, or skull. It is called the "*dura mater*," meaning "hard mother" or "tough mother" in Latin. This membrane is tough and waterproof. It attaches to most of the skull bones, divides the skull into compartments; it also lines the spinal column. The *dura mater* also protects more delicate membranes inside the skull. (The term is commonly abbreviated by using the word "dura" as a shorter way of saying "*dura mater*.") Let's be very clear about one point: this tissue—the dura—is directly attached to the bone of the skull. Because of this connection, if the skull is tilted and twisted inside, the dura will follow those twists and turns as surely as the stripe down the middle of a highway follows that road.

If all the dura did was to divide the skull into compartments like the sections of a grapefruit, it wouldn't be so extraordinary. However, the dura covers, surrounds, attaches to, penetrates or influences every nerve, organ, blood vessel and bone in the entire body! The dura is continuous in the front of the head with the coverings of the optic nerves and the sclera or white of the eye, thus it can affect vision. Commonly while a person is undergoing a Bio Cranial procedure, his or her sight will brighten and sharpen. Colors will appear more vivid; depth perception and night vision often improve. The dura also surrounds the pituitary gland and under the wrong circumstances can put pressure on the gland and its blood supply. This can dramatically alter hormone balance.

I had a thirty-year-old female patient who had a benign thyroid tumor. She had stopped having menstrual periods and her hair was thinning. She also had an extremely high blood sugar level of 250. If your random blood sugar is less than 100 mg/dL (100 <u>milligrams</u> per <u>decilitre</u>—5.55 mmol/L), it's normal. This is a blood sugar level taken without regard to when you had a meal or snack containing calories. Any level higher than 200 would suggest diabetes. She had also had had low back surgery, but was still in pain. Unfortunately this is all too common. She informed me that she was diabetic, and I told her I would only work on her if she promised to monitor her blood sugar level. I asked her to do this because we have seen many cases of high blood sugar levels dropping after a Bio Cranial Procedure.

I didn't see her for another two and a half months because she lived very far from my office. With just the one treatment, her blood sugar had dropped to 115, her menstrual period came back, her tumor shrank, and her hair was growing in thicker. She had much less pain in her lower back and wanted relief for that and after her second visit it disappeared!

Why would these hormone imbalances respond to Bio Cranial Therapy? It occurred partly because we were able to get the dura to stop pulling on and squeezing the pituitary inside the skull. But why did her back get better, even though she had already had back surgery that failed?

The dura leaves the head through a large hole in the occiput (the back, bottom bone in the skull). It directly attaches into the top two cervical vertebrae (neck bones)—the atlas and the axis. When these two vertebrae become misaligned, chiropractors know the patient will have trouble. The blood supply to the brain arrives through the right and left vertebral arteries, and these arteries travel through holes in the side of each of the seven cervical vertebrae. Twisting of these vertebrae can alter the blood flow. This can, in turn, create fatigue, dizziness, high blood pressure, and especially headaches. It can also affect the pituitary gland and other brain structures. Vital spinal nerves are also influenced in an adverse way. A misaligned second vertebra will interfere with neck rotation, and can also lead to dysfunction in the eyes, ears, tongue, forehead and sinuses.

The dura also forms "sleeves" covering all of the spinal nerve roots from top to bottom. If the dura has a pull on it from distortions in the arrangement of the head bones, so will these sleeves. In addition, the dura directly attaches into the sacrum—a spade-shaped bone at the base of the spine—and the coccyx or "tailbone." The release of tension that Bio Cranial correction affords allows the low back to realign itself, stopping the irritation of the nerves that cause pain and organ problems. Chiropractors have been right about the importance of good spinal alignment. The brain and the body "talk to each other" through the nerves; we want the "call" to go through clearly, rather than like a static-filled cell phone call during a thunderstorm. Why continue to reposition (adjust) the neck and low back repeatedly (as chiropractors do) if the dura is able to pull all of the vertebrae right back into their old positions? The remedy is simple—correct the head instead!

So, what is a "reciprocal tension membrane system"? This system works like this: you have this tough tissue attaching to the inside of the skull on one end (like the large dog I talked about on the leash), and everything else in the body is on the other end of the leash (again, like in the example given earlier about my trying to pull the leash on the dog to go visit my friend). In most people, the leash is very tight all the time. The question is: Do you exhaust yourself fighting with the dog and risk getting bitten, or would you rather be the loving master the dog wants and needs, and be happy together?

The Bio Cranial System is Born

Dr. Boyd wasn't the first doctor to believe that the cranium has clinical significance. The notion that the cranial bones move first appeared in 1905. It was the inspiration of William Garner Sutherland, an early osteopathic student. This has since been confirmed in primate studies.

Unfortunately, most doctors mistakenly believe that the cranial bones are fused. Why—Gray's *Anatomy*. No, not the sexy Sunday night television show—Henry Gray's British tome on the structure of the human body, *Anatomy of the Human Body*. The confusion arises because there are (surprise!) differences between living people and dead people—cadavers. Gray's *Anatomy* was based on his study of cadavers. In a cadaver, the cartilage between the various sections of the skull turns to glue, and obliterates the space between the cranial bones. This gives the understandably erroneous impression of a fused skull. However, in a living human being, the bones are living and moving tissue, there is space between the skull plates that is maintained by the cartilage, and the bones open and close continuously in rhythmic fashion. This movement is essential for healthy human functioning. Classical osteopathy in the cranial Field first received some positive attention in the 1950s.

Around 1970, Dr. Boyd was practicing in Ireland, specializing in a type of herbal medicine. He received an invitation to attend a two-year post-graduate training program in cranial osteopathy in London. For a long time, he'd had an intuition the cranium was a major key in terms of helping the body to correct itself (more on this later). His teacher, Professor Dennis Brookes, taught a more classical version of cranial osteopathy which was subtle, slow, and for Dr. Boyd, quite frustrating. He did ignite a spark when he said to this elite class: "You know, there's really only one disease." Everyone in the class leaned forward to hear what the great man was going to say. Professor Brookes finished his thought with one term: "over-contraction."

Dr. Boyd approached this word the way a Zen student would a koan—a teaching riddle—given by the Master (teacher). What did it mean? What was over-contracted, and what could one do about it? Space does not allow me to elaborate on the mental process Dr. Boyd went through. At the end of it all, however, he knew his teacher meant over-contraction of the entire cranio-sacral system. This gave rise to his understanding that we have a stressed system already stressed, just waiting for some minor stress to come along and tip us over the edge and exhibit symptoms of distress. He understood that the skull pulls on the dura, the dura pulls on everything else and we get into trouble throughout the body. We then start looking for answers in all the wrong places.

In allopathic medicine, chiropractic, and other healing arts, we are taught to look at pieces of things. In medicine, we look at symptoms and how to alleviate them primarily through drugs that force something in the body to change. The whole field of medicine has become specialized, with doctors doing residencies in smaller and smaller areas of specialization. In chiropractic, we adjust twenty-four individual spinal segments in addition to some extra-spinal areas to realign the spine and help the nerves. We have charts in our offices showing which vertebrae and spinal nerves are associated with which organs and symptoms. Acupuncturists use needling and other techniques to change the flow of energy in the body. They study twelve major "meridians" plus their inner pathways and eight extra meridians. (For the uninitiated, meridians are the twelve major channels that run up and down the body. In traditional Asian medicine, meridians are believed to carry *chi*—a vital substance in the body. One of the central concepts of acupuncture is that points along these meridians can be used to restore proper function to their corresponding systems or organs.) Dr. Boyd calls this a "segmental approach" to healing.

The BCS is not segmental in its nature or approach—it is global. Going back to Archimedes, we are moving the world by using the proper leverage. Rather than forcing the segments to change, we are helping the body reorganize itself on a global level—throughout the entire body—changing all of its segments through one skillfully applied movement. Rather than moving one or several vertebrae manually, or giving one or several medicines for a constellation of symptoms, we seek to eliminate the root of the problem. This corrective movement is applied on each side of the head assisting the cranium in opening like a bud on a tree in springtime. The body's entire level of functioning miraculously improves as a result. Isn't nature wonderful?

When my family and I moved from New York to Texas in late 2003, I opened a new practice. Because I had been involved with Bio Cranial now for several years and was an instructor for the Bio Cranial Institute, I decided to call my new practice "Head to Foot."

One day, I met a lady at a lecture I was giving. Ilean Irwin had pain in the heels of both feet bad enough to warrant cortisone shots. As you might imagine, she had been given all kinds of advice about her feet and shoes. The pain had continued for six years, despite the periodic shots which merely took the edge off her pain for a short time. Did I work on her feet? No—I worked on her head. The pain left, and to this day has never come back. It certainly justified the name of my clinic!

Dr. Boyd's radical approach is to focus on the "predisposing" level of cause—over-contracted dura rather than the precipitating or triggering factors. He looks at the whole system and the universal source of stress that gives everyone a tendency to develop one type of physical problem or another. If someone came to see him with knee pain or learning disabilities (the head *certainly* might be a factor there, duh!), he would relate it back to the head. Because of our different understanding and approach to the body, Certified Bio Cranial Practitioners around the globe routinely get results where results have been slow to appear before. How can we get it right so often? Why?

The Bio Cranial Solution: *You* are the Miracle You've Been Looking For!

Do you have to be a genius or have special abilities to administer Bio Cranial corrections? Fortunately for me, you don't. You just have to be a good student. The reason that medical doctors, chiropractors, osteopaths, and acupuncturists (forgive me if I have left your profession out and you assume it belongs here) have ever gotten *any* therapeutic result is that the body is designed to be self-regulating and self-healing. Our aliveness and awareness is always present, even as the body is forming. It wants to express itself in a healthy and comfortable way. This inborn—innate—tendency toward health and balance is called "homeostasis" in the medical physiology books.

Each healing art discipline has its own terminology, but one of the things we all agree on is that the body has some type of intelligence guiding its internal functioning. We know how to grow from a single cell at conception into a very complex human organism. We generally can grow two eyes on the front of the head and two ears on each side, instead of the other way around. Go ahead and call that genetics if it makes you happy. I believe there is more to our physiology than can be fully explained by what we now call "science."

What happens that gets us into all this trouble we call "pain" and "sickness"? We have systems that are functioning under the load of stress. Aren't there such factors as emotional stress, toxicity, and nutritional deficiency? Of course there are. And all of these are intensified and aggravated by the predisposing level of cause that Dr. Boyd has learned to respect and manage—over-contraction of the cranio-sacral system.

Why is this such a universal problem? Our heads are out of shape and the bones are pulling on the dura, and the dura is pulling on everything else! Why are the twenty-two bones of the head in poor alignment with one another? Obviously, head injuries from sports and accidents can cause them to shift and lock into bad positions.

However, we also see children and even infants with major cranial imbalances along with the impairments they cause. Food for thought: How does modern birthing contribute to the troubles we face as senior citizens (and not-so-senior citizens)? The use of forceps, suction, and episiotomies can contribute to the infant's soft head getting out of shape. C-Sections—cesarean sections—are not necessarily gentle or easy by nature, and they inhibit the expansion of the cranial bones that normally takes place as the baby's head exits the birth canal. The compression and expansion of the head during a "normal" birth starts the cycle of normal cranial movement that we talked about earlier. More food for thought: What if the mother's pelvis is twisted while the baby's head is forming? Obviously we'd need at least a whole other chapter to discuss these issues with any depth.

My Dream and Heart's Desire

At the beginning of this chapter, I stated that I believed I had received a rich inheritance. My dream and heart's desire is to pass that inheritance onto you. What would it be like if no child had to wear a back brace for scoliosis, or (worse) have Harrington Rods surgically inserted to support his or her spine? What would it be like for older people to regain their sense of balance and safety when walking, as many of our stroke patients have done? And what would it be like if people could reduce their need for medication, because they no longer needed it? Thousands of people walk, run and bicycle to raise money for research with the hope of finding medical cures for various diseases. Is this research generally leading to an improved quality of life for people, or are we continuing to pour money into bottomless holes while we ignore a monumental discovery that is already gathering clinical proof that it works?

Bio Cranial Research

Although the Bio Cranial Institute is still small, we are working to publish articles in reputable scientific journals. Documented case histories are being submitted by many of our member doctors. Establishing Bio Cranial Therapy has helped patients with Type one and Type two diabetes, fibromyalgia, post-surgical pain and many other conditions. We have a research director who determines which research papers meet the strict criteria needed for submission to journals. During the next few years, look for more information coming out in the scientific journals and the media about the Bio Cranial System.

More Information about The Bio Cranial System

The Bio Cranial Institute has established a website: www.biocranial.com. There is also ample information available at www.drstuart.net. After an introductory page featuring a welcome by Dr. Boyd, this web site is divided into a section for patients and a section for practitioners. The patient side includes introductory material explaining the Bio Cranial System and a search engine for finding a Bio Cranial practitioner near you, if a properly trained doctor is available in your locale.

If you know of (or perhaps you are) a chiropractor, medical or osteopathic physician, naturopath, dentist, or acupuncturist who would be a good candidate to learn and apply this most powerful system, he/she or you should visit the practitioner side of the website. My e-mail address for doctors is: dr.marmorstein@biocranial.com. Patient inquiries should be addressed to: contact@drstuart.net or to the Bio Cranial website.

Welcome to the Bio Cranial universe, and may you find the health, freedom, and happiness you seek.

About The Author

Dr. Stuart C. Marmorstein

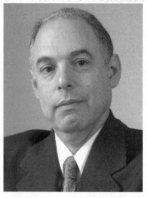

Dr. Stuart C. Marmorstein has been involved with the healing arts since high school, when he had 3 National Science Foundation grants for summer study. One grant was for a Bioscience program in Philadelphia's Hahnemann Hospital. He was exposed to laboratory and clinical research, and also worked in the ER and Intensive Care Unit. Before graduation, he was already accepted into the Jefferson Medical College as well as into The Pennsylvania State University, where he got a B.A. in Psychology. While impressed with medicine's successes in crisis care, his interest shifted toward how we can restore and maintain health naturally. He graduated from Texas Chiropractic College in 1979, and has since practiced in Texas and New York. He spent 2 years in India doing chiropractic relief work. Dr. Marmorstein has taught post-graduate classes since 1979, and now specializes in Dr. Robert Boyd's Bio Cranial System. He is the Executive Vice President of the Bio Cranial Institute and is one of its senior instructors. "Dr. Stuart" is coauthor of a case study on Bio Cranial and fibromyalgia. He speaks to lay and professional audiences around the US about the powerful relationship between the bones of the head and optimum health.

Stuart C. Marmorstein, D.C.
Executive Vice President, The Bio Cranial Institute
Managing Director, Head to Foot, LLC
Phone: 936.494.HEAD (4323) / Conroe Office
Phone: 713.831.6875 / Houston Office
Phone: 281.838.4328 / Bio Cranial Institute
Fax: 775.254.2757
Email: contact@drstuart.net / dr.marmorstein@biocranial.com
www.drstuart.net / www.biocranial.com

Chapter 11

The Elusive Self-Esteem Gene: The Paradigm Shift from Self-Loathing to Self-Love

Dr. Helene B. Leonetti

No one can make you feel inferior without your consent.
—Eleanor Roosevelt

What if, each day upon waking, we asked ourselves the question: "What must I do today to fall deeply in love with myself?" Debbie Ford posed this question in a workshop I attended, and it caused a palpable pause in the room as we all mused the profound significance of its meaning.

When, in our entire lives, have we *ever* asked that question? What we do ask is more like, "What must I do to make him love me," or "What must I do for them to approve of me?" Self-love is the genesis of self-esteem, and yet we have permitted the outer culture to lobotomize us with the idea that service to others is the byword.

Let me tell you a story. I am a very successful holistic gynecologist who came up from the position of practicing nursing for twenty years before entering medical school. For the past ten years, I have gained fame in the research world with my clinical trials using transdermal progesterone cream for hormone balance. And my colleagues, who at first dubbed me the local "quack," are now coming around to respecting my expertise in the world of herbs and bioidentical hormones—interesting ducks, we doctors.

Finally out of my third toxic marriage, I am settled in, happily living with my precious cat, Shadow, and starting that long over-due love affair with myself.

Well, eight weeks ago, I awoke with swollen, red, itchy eyes, and sought help from one of my family practice buddies, thinking it an allergic dermatitis. Five specialists, an herbalist, and two psychics later, I am humbled to say that this is all a soul issue. Oh, do not diminish the physical implications of such origins: my cornea became inflamed, and I am looking at everyone as if I am underwater, feeling like someone has thrown gravel in my eyes. Being a gynecologist and looking into deep dark holes all day long does not help.

What has emerged from this challenge, affirming over and over again is that *every* physical malady always bubbles up from the soul. My inability to "see" certain aspects of myself was the genesis. When God wants to get our attention, it must be some-thing we are forced to look at. A bothersome rash on a leg is too easily covered so we can ignore it and continue with our dysfunc-tion.

Our journey in this incarnation is to be the best that we can be, physically, emotionally, intellectually, and spiritually. Being ruthlessly honest with who we are is essential for this journey. Yet we all carry baggage from our past that interferes with this precious journey. My sadness and guilt about making so many unhealthy choices—especially in intimate relationships—are be-ing pushed up from the deep recesses of my soul, and forced into my vision for forgiveness and healing.

Yet we prostitute ourselves to stay in material comfort, despite a toxic relationship. And the irony of life is that some of us stay beaten and broken, others become closed of heart and hopelessly cynical; yet, some of us fight to thrive and become strong and em-powered. What makes this diversity—this distinction in our response to traumas in the outside world? It is *self-esteem*.

My beloved teacher and mentor, Deepak Chopra, calls what happens when we become lobotomized to buy into the cultural beliefs—"socially programmed hypnosis." And make no mistake; this is a powerful force to reckon with. Some of our magnificent visionaries were killed or driven to suicide because their beliefs and teachings threatened the status quo: Galileo, Socrates, Semmelweis (who described childbirth sepsis which killed hundreds of thousands of new mothers because the doctors were too arrogant to wash their hands between deliveries).

When people like Thoreau, Emerson, and even our contemporary Chopra, speak their truths, they are often disparaged and mocked for their far-reaching views of how we exist in our universe. I have plagiarized Deepak's teaching that "our birthright is perfect health," not disease, and that our thoughts create our reality. In fact, one just has to quote the Bible, as well as all the great sages and prophets who ever lived, to remind ourselves that, "as a man thinketh, so is he"—Proverbs 23:7. Wayne Dyer reminds us to put our attention on what we desire, not on what we do not want.

The recently released movie, *What The Bleep Do We Know!?*™ entertains us while teaching how quantum physics and spirituality are connected. Our thoughts actually *do* create our reality, and in fact, we alter our very cellular tissue with our thoughts—stinking thinking makes sick cells. And after understanding how the molecular configuration of water can be symmetrical and beautiful when surrounded with loving thoughts, and distorted and ugly with hateful thoughts, imagine what we do to our bodies, which are comprised of at least seventy percent water!

We have been programmed to believe that everyone is more important than we are. The three megalithic establishments cement this teaching. Organized religion tells us we are sinners, and God will punish us; corporate America has shown us that belief in the integrity of financial wizards is naïve; and conventional medicine is hell bent on keeping us victims in a system that foists its authoritarianism over us, forgetting that empowerment through education is a win-win situation.

As Ram Das says, "When you are in love, its like going into a tub. Come Into love." And all this talk is really about "self-love" without which we cannot love someone else. For in fact, we are *all* one—when I love me, I love God, for God and I are one, so now I can love you and now you and I and God are one, not one jot separated from each other.

The ego is that little leprechaun sitting on your left shoulder yapping about how stupid you are and how ugly and how useless.

When we are foolish enough to believe it, we actually *become* stupid, ugly, and useless.

That negative ego edges God out then gleefully dances about, knowing he got yet another victim to believe that all that is, is outside us and seeable; but in fact, all that matters is what is *inside*. Shakespeare knew what he was doing when he wrote, "Go to your bosom; knock there and ask your heart what it doth know."—*Measure for Measure* by William Shakespeare.

When a patient comes in, I remind her not to slump, sitting there as if she were invisible. "Shoulders back, chest out, head high,' I tell her. And I evoke the image of beautiful Audrey Hepburn—that gracious lady who would walk into a room and everyone would turn to look at her.

Self-esteem is not earned—it is accepted. You are unique and unrepeatable, and no one can perform your divine mission. One of my favorite "fierce Goddesses," Clarissa Pinkola Estés, author of, *Women Who Run with the Wolves*, has this to say about purpose, "...One of the most calming and powerful actions you can do to intervene in a stormy world is to stand up and show your soul. Soul on deck shines like gold in dark times. The light of the soul throws sparks, can send up flares, builds signal fires...causes proper matters to catch fire. To display the lantern of soul in shadowy times like these—to be fierce and to show mercy toward others, both—are acts of immense bravery and greatest necessity. Struggling souls catch light from other souls who are fully lit and willing to show it. If you would help to calm the tumult, this is one of the strongest things you can do.

"...There will always be times in the midst of 'success right around the corner, but as yet still unseen' when you feel discouraged. I too have felt despair many times in my life, but I do not keep a chair for it; I will not entertain it. It is not allowed to eat from my plate. The reason is this: In my uttermost bones I know something, as do you. It is that there can be no despair when you remember why you came to Earth, who you serve, and who sent you here. The good words we say and the good deeds we do are not ours: They are the words and deeds of the One who brought us here. In that spirit, I hope you will write this on your wall: When a great ship is in harbor and moored, it is safe, there can be no doubt. But...that is not what great ships are built for.

"...This comes with much love and prayer that you remember who you came from and why you came to this beautiful, needful Earth."

A prime responsibility for nursing students was to assist interns during special procedures. One patient with meningitis was scheduled for a spinal tap—a technique for removing spinal fluid from the lower back through a needle. The intern was using Novocain to numb the area where the needle would be inserted.

This intern, a tall, dark-haired Armenian chap, affable and conscientious, asked me to gather the necessary equipment. I ran to several different spots to retrieve the goods. For some quirky reason the tiny glass ampoules of Novocaine were sitting in a little plastic container alongside a potent medication called Levophed, used when a patient is in shock. Not only is this drug very concentrated, requiring dilution before being administered intravenously, but there is a bold warning on the drug insert page to prevent this medication, at all costs, from entering the subcutaneous tissue beneath the surface of the skin; it could cause a profound decrease in blood supply to that area, resulting in gangrene.

You guessed it: instead of grabbing the pain numbing Novocaine, I got the Levophed. Then ignoring Rule number one—to always check medications carefully before administering—we went ahead. As the doctor was injecting our unsuspecting patient, I remember him wincing and complaining of discomfort. Our poor patient was having a dangerous drug injected into the soft tissue of his back, and it wasn't until the tap was completed that I discovered my grievous error. I shook in stark terror at my mistake. Pale and shaking, I crept in to see the doctor and confess my deed. That handsome face became chalky white and little beads of sweat immediately broke out on his upper lip. He didn't yell at me, as certainly I deserved, but instructed me to keep watch on the patient throughout the night. We made out an "Incident Report," which is a medico-legal requirement, but didn't let our patient know about the mistake. How I agonized throughout that night and how I prayed to God to forgive me. Fortunately, this young man suffered no ill effects. You can imagine my profound relief and gratitude. What a way to learn a lesson!

The summer before I entered nursing school, I went to Cape Cod with some high school buddies. Staying in the Buccaneer Motel in Provincetown, Massachusetts, we met some lovely chaps from Pennsylvania. Herbert was my personal choice, and we maintained a correspondence by mail for six months at which time he invited me to a New Year's Eve party in his hometown, Philly.

What follows is a glimpse into the emotional frailty and tottering self-esteem that I would carry with me for the next twenty-five years.

In preparation for my momentous date with the desirable Herbert, my mother had sewn me a magnificent dress. It was a jewel-green velvet-skirted number topped with spaghetti-strapped mint-green brocade. It was gorgeous! And I was mightily excited.

I had always been blessed with beautiful, flawless skin. But just days before New Year's Eve, I was graced with the appearance of twenty-one pimples on my face, one for each year I lived on the planet. Now I was devastated! But with the help of some makeup, I was able to cover it up successfully. I boarded a train in my green confection, and, if I do say so myself, looked fairly well turned out—beautiful, in fact. Herb greeted me at the train station with a look, I noted, of instant approval.

If it had been at all within my power, I would have pulled that night off with great success. But it seems that was not to be. My miserable self-esteem surfaced, and for some reason I can't even explain, I felt compelled to explain to each and every person present that night the story of my pimple breakout. The entire evening, of course, was a disaster—irreparable—and I never heard from Herb again.

My self-esteem wouldn't improve much as time went on. Later, as a nurse I was bound and determined to find "Mr. Right." I longed for a "true love" relationship and would sit with my best friend night after night in a restaurant near the hospital staring at various medical student possibilities, each one of whom I was convinced would become my soul mate. Most of these guys I had neither met nor even talked to, but I still fantasized about becoming involved in a meaningful, heart-stopping relationship. This need I had to be known and loved would follow me through many years of searching until finally one day I became enlightened to the knowledge that it was actually my own self—*me*—from whom I wanted to know love and acceptance.

When I was eighteen I went to my high school guidance counselor and asked, "What should I be?"

To which she answered, "You are a woman; you can become a nurse, or a teacher."

Nice and simple...and constricting. Nobody suggested I could become an aeronautical engineer, lawyer, doctor, physicist or racecar driver; my options were only two: nurse or teacher. Having no mentor to challenge my choice and seeing no other option, I entered nursing school.

Being told at the age of eighteen that my gender allowed for so few career choices, however noble they may have been, in retrospect was a gift because a germinal seed was planted which would lead to a wonderful personal evolution. I would have stayed a nurse, but for the mass cultural mindset that demands respect and attention be paid to the physician. Wanting that same respect and attention for myself pushed me toward attaining my M.D. degree.

My self-esteem and self-assuredness, however, lagged miserably behind my goal setting. And the nursing environment from which I was emerging certainly was no help; the nursing structure never supported the idea that we nurses were anything more than second-class citizens. I remember being instructed to stand and offer my chair to his highness, the doctor, when he entered the room.

Even despite my long uphill climb to achieve what appeared to be an enviable position, I continued to feel inadequate, allowing the mean little voice inside to taunt me, reminding me how stupid and ill-prepared I was. During the darkest days of my depression, I remember lying in bed, sleepless, forcing myself to go through the steps of surgically performing a vaginal hysterectomy—a formidable task for me as this area of gynecological surgery was the one in which I was the most poorly taught. That little niggling ego continued its taunts and jeers at my inadequacy, wearing down my defenses, and more importantly, eroding the kernel of self-esteem that represented my identity to the world. As a result, every flaw and every weakness in my knowledge, I wore pathetically on my sleeve for the world to see and exploit.

We are all mirror images of each other, so that when I think I am less than perfect, so also does every friend and stranger I meet. Menopause often brings to the surface of our lives many of the insecurities, perceived "failings," and little secrets we have tucked away into the farthest depths of our soul. For so long throughout our lives we have ignored them, believing they might simply go away. But in this magical time of menopause, we are privileged to get to know these aspects of ourselves. Privileged, you ask? Yes, because they provide keys to our true nature from which satisfaction and fulfillment emerge.

The examining room is where I share what I call "sacred dialogue." My conversations with patients demand that I be present—truly present—and for that I must take care of myself first. Sometimes it isn't easy fitting in all the aspects of nurturing my physical, emotional, and spiritual requirements, but I make time anyway.

The first thing on my agenda, after feeding my magnificent cat, Shadow, is meditation. If I don't start my day with deep breathing, prayer, and an attitude of gratitude (all of which takes about twenty minutes), I can feel fragmented, scattered, and most importantly, not present. I must be *with* you to hear your story so we can work together to mastermind a plan.

I am struck by how conditioned women are—the minute they enter my examining room, they get on the table, lie down, and spread their legs.

"Wait a minute," I say, "I want to look at *all* of you, not just your pelvis!"

Then I lighten them up with the following scenario: "Imagine a CEO, well-dressed in an impeccably cut Italian suit, entering an examination room. In walks a gorgeous female urologist. Without any further ado, the CEO unbuckles his trousers, drops his drawers, and bends over to receive his prostate check. Can you just imagine that?"

We laugh and now you may be wondering what all this has to do with self-esteem. Well, it's subtle, but think about it. We women have been allowing medical doctors to have their way with us without their knowing or caring who we are. Not great for the self-esteem, eh? There is much more to you than your pelvis. Unfortunately, the super-specialists think that only "their part" counts.

When I consider the entire human being, I learn so much about them. Along with the "human connection" of actually looking an individual in the eye, I can tell much by simply scanning the outer body. For example, dry brittle hair might signal thyroid dysfunction or hormone imbalance or a lack of essential minerals and essential fatty acids. Reddened eyes can hint at problems ranging from sleeplessness and anemia to poor-fitting contact lenses. I even diagnosed one woman as having AIDS because she exhibited a thrush on a throat exam (white spots caused by a fungus).

What is so pervasive in conversations with my fellow goddesses is their lack of self-acceptance, lack of self-esteem, and lack of self-love. I usually begin these talks with the question, "Are you healthy?"

The answers I get back are mostly self-deprecating. "I'm healthy, but I'm fat," or, "I'm healthy, but I'm not exercising as I should," or, "I'm healthy, but I'm eating all the wrong things." Sometimes I feel as if I'm in a confessional complete with clerical collar, listening to the sinful unburden themselves. What I wouldn't give to hear one of you say, "I'm healthy, happy, and satisfied with myself just as I am. I just want to make a few minor adjustments."

Louise Hay is a brilliant metaphysical lecturer and teacher, and I offer thanks to Jill Kramer at Hay House for letting me reprint this excerpt from Louise's book, *Gratitude: A Way of Life*.

> *I have noticed that the Universe loves gratitude. The more grateful you are, the more goodies you get. When I say "goodies," I don't mean only material things. I mean all the people, places and experiences that make life so wonderfully worth living. You know how great you feel when your life is filled with love and joy and health and creativity, and you get the green lights and the parking places. This is how our lives are meant to be lived. The Universe is a generous, abundant giver, and it likes to be appreciated.*
>
> *Gratitude brings more to be grateful about. It increases your abundant life. Lack of gratitude or complaining, brings little to rejoice about. Complainers always find that they have little good in their life, or they do no enjoy what they do have. The Universe always gives us what we believe we deserve. Many of us have been raised to look at what we do not have and to feel only lack. We come from a belief in scarcity, and wonder why our lives are so empty. If we believe that "I don't have, and I won't be happy until I do..." then we are putting our lives on hold. What the Universe hears is: "I*

don't have, and I am not happy," and that is what you get more of.

When I awaken in the morning, the first thing I do before I even open my eyes is to thank my bed for a good night's sleep. I am grateful for the warmth and comfort it has given me. From the beginning, it is easy to think of many, many more things that I am grateful for. By the time I have gotten out of bed, I have probably expressed gratitude for 80 to 100 people, places, things, and experiences in my life. This is a great way to start the day.

In the evening, just before sleep, I go through the day, blessing and being grateful for each experience. I also forgive myself if I feel that I made a mistake, or said something inappropriate, or made decisions that was not the best. This exercise fills me with warm fuzzies and I drift off to sleep like a happy baby.

We even want to be grateful for the lessons we have. Don't run from lessons: they are little packages of treasures that have been given to us. As we learn from them, our lives change for the better. I now rejoice whenever I see another portion of the dark side of myself. I know that it means that I am ready to let go of something that has been hindering my life. I say, "thank you for showing me this, so I can heal it and move on." So whether the lesson is a "problem" that has cropped up or an opportunity to see an old, negative pattern within us that it is time to let go of, rejoice!"

There is so much wisdom in that passage—our thoughts *do* create our reality—so if we are always complaining about what we don't have instead of blessing what we do, we just keep ourselves in the mire of despair. That is why I stress over and over that we must love ourselves as we are. We are all jewels in the making—works in progress. The phrase,*"you can look at the glass as either half empty or half full,"* may seem trite, but it is profound in its meaning.

Martyrdom is pathological and actually quite harmful to loved ones who might be receiving our constant care. When our children witness our harried demeanor and seething resentment about always being on call for them, they may well get the notion that motherhood stinks. Why not give your child the gift of witnessing you taking care of *your* needs. That implicitly gives *them* permission to nurture themselves, and the sick pathological cycle of martyrdom will at last be broken.

One of the most toxic attitudes we have originates inside our own heads. Have you ever received a compliment, then said, "Yeah, but—" Patrick Collard is a master intuitive and body worker, who has developed a tape series called *Success Without Sabotage,* in which he speaks of our inability to love self by "yeah, butting" everything. We need simply say, "T*hank you,*" and then give ourselves a hug.

For years we have entertained images of ourselves as second-class citizens. After all, we just got the vote a mere eighty years ago. Women in certain third world countries still walk ten paces behind their men folk, and they hide their magnificent curls from the outside world. In certain countries male children are considered superior to female, and women are still aborting themselves if ultrasound reveals a female fetus in order to avoid losing their dowry or even their lives.

Even though in America we have legislated equality, we remain toxic in our thinking, buying in to all the teaching of our inferiority.

So my precious sisters, I want you practice something special each and every day, four times. Practice this in front of a mirror which is so much more powerful: Look yourself in the eye—the looking glass into the soul—and say out loud the following, "*I [your name], I accept you, I appreciate you, I forgive you, and I love you, exactly as you are.*"

About The Author

Dr. Helene B. Leonetti

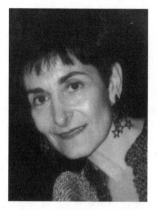

My 45-year odyssey from nurse to doctor to healer and beyond began in 1961. Being given two choices, nurse or teacher, simplified my path: nursing consumed my passion to nurture, but being a physician gave me the power to help fashion how we engage our patients in the process of healing. The intervening years between then and now witnessed my growth into being a holistic physician, being board certified now not only as an Obstetrician-Gynecologist, but also as a Founding Diplomat of the American Board of Holistic Medicine. My study with master herbalist, David Winston, has rounded off my knowledge of herbs and nutrition to provide a comprehensive program for my patients. Thirteen years ago, I met my beloved mentor and colleague, John R. Lee, MD., who ignited my passion and enthusiasm for natural transdermal proges- terone, the bio-identical form of one of the two important female hormones creating balance and harmony in our bodies. Shortly after meeting John, I began a research trial that was to demonstrate signifi- cant improvement over the placebo of hot flashes, experienced by the women in menopause. Two subsequent studies proving uterine protec- tiveness when used with estrogen have been published, and I began my fourth, and final trial, intending to show bone protectiveness in women 70 years and beyond. I presently practice office gynecology in Bethlehem, PA, and lecture widely. My book *Menopause: A Spiritual Renaissance* is a culmination of my life's work.

Dr. Helene B. Leonetti
Email: littlelion1@verizon.net
www.helenbeleonettimd.com

Special Feature

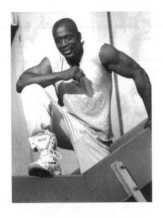

David Wright Interviews
Billy Blanks
Creator of Tae Bo®

Chapter 12

Billy Blanks

THE INTERVIEW

David E. Wright (Wright)

Today we are talking with Billy Blanks, one of the most sought-after trainers and fitness consultants in the world. He has earned a seventh-degree black belt in Tae Kwon Do, as well as black belts in five other forms of martial arts. He is a seven-time Karate champion and has won thirty-six gold medals in international competition. In 1975, he became the first Amateur Athletic Union Karate Champion, a title he held for five consecutive years. In 1980, he was selected as captain of the U.S. Karate Team, and in 1994 he won the Massachusetts Golden Glove championship in the light heavyweight class and the Tri-State Golden Glove Champion of Champions.

Billy has appeared in more than twenty action films and is a popular guest in television series. His books and videos are among the best selling in the world. Billy Blanks, welcome to *A Healthier You*.

Billy Blanks (Blanks)

Well, thanks, for having me. I'm glad to be here.

Wright

Great. You know, it's hard to imagine that you were the fourth of fifteen children, were born with a medical condition that kept you out of sports, struggled through school, and then were diagnosed with dyslexia at the age of 37. Look at where you are today! How in the world did you make it?

Blanks

Well, I actually believe it's a blessing. I thank God for being able to do the things I'm doing right now, because if it wasn't for Him, I wouldn't be able to actually sit here and talk to you on the phone. He has given me strength and power in knowing that I can endure and be better and more than I thought I could be. It's an awesome thing.

Wright

What was the medical condition?

Blanks

Well, one was my tendons—I did not have flexibility in my body. Some people are born with tight tendons and muscle tissue, and the doctors said I would never be flexible. But I studied skeletons and the human body and read about muscle tissue. Then, I thought, "Well if you took the muscle off the body, the skeleton can go anywhere, no matter whose body it is." So, I began to stretch every day, and I forced myself into being able to endure the pain regarding my flexibility. Then the next thing I knew, I started gaining flexibility—my body started to become flexible— muscles started to relax, and I started to learn how to put oxygen into muscle and blood so I could learn how to relax my body. From there flexibility started coming. Now, I can do any kind of split, any kind of stretch or anything a ballet dancer, or a martial arts person needs to do to make himself or herself better or to become a better puncher or kicker.

Wright

Without pain?

Blanks

Without pain. Now, I can do a full straddle. When you look at my muscle structure, you wouldn't think I was that flexible, but I can do a full straddle down, and I can do the "cheerleader split." A long time ago I couldn't do that. It took me the know-how and the will to want to push myself to where the doctor told me I couldn't go.

If you let somebody tell you that you'll never be able to achieve certain things, then you won't go try them and you won't do them. I didn't accept what I was told I couldn't do. I just worked hard at it, and eventually I started to see progress. And, when improvement started to appear, the next thing I knew I could say, "Wow! If I can do *that,* then I can to *this.*" It's just awesome to know you can do anything you want to do if you just put your mind and heart to it.

Wright

Billy, you work very closely with your wife, Gayle, and your teenage daughter, Shelly, who is also a Karate champion. Your son, Billy, Jr., is a singer and dancer in Los Angeles. Did your parents instill family values in you?

Blanks

Yes. I grew up in a family where my father always told us that in order for us to get anything out of life, we're going have to work for it because nobody is ever going to give us anything for nothing. He always taught us that discipline and focus was the key to being successful in life. We needed to work, we needed to share things, and we needed to love each other. Growing up in a big family—growing up with all those brothers and sisters—we learned how to share. We had to wear each other's shoes, and we had to play with each other's toys because we couldn't afford to have individual toys for ourselves. We learned those things beginning as young kids. We also learned how to fight—you know, kids are always going to argue. I would never say we were perfect kids, but our mother and father showed us a lot of love.

Our parents showed us so much love I didn't even know I was poor. We lived in a poor neighborhood, but my father and mother always made sure our needs were met. Through the grace of God, we were blessed to be able to have a mother who loved Jesus Christ and a father who loved Jesus Christ. That kept us and nourished us as young kids.

Wright

My brother had seven children and, even now that he's gone, we kids stay together. You'd think a big family like ours would scatter to the four corners of the earth, but no matter where we go, we are very, very close.

Now, let's talk about your foundation. Since you personally donated a million dollars to establish it, you must be serious about it.

Blanks

Yes, I *am* serious about it. Others helped me get to where I needed to go to be able to do the things I've done in my life and, in view of that, I determined that if I got the opportunity I would give back. Now, since God has given me the opportunity to establish a foundation, I think it's truly a blessing to go out and help the needy.

Wright

Your stated mission at the foundation is to equip high-risk women and children with life skills to achieve their full potential and then give back to society. How does the foundation do that?

Blanks

Well, Winifred goes around and looks at various women-of-need programs. We then determine where we can help out in that program, and if we can help, we will fund the program. We'll give them things we would like to see them do within the confines of our foundation, to help them reach their goals. Our goal is not to give anything away but to teach people how to "fish." Do you know what I mean?

Wright

Oh, yes.

Blanks

Because, if we teach a person how to do something, then they can go out in the world and become successful, but if you just give them something and not give them the knowledge and the ability to overcome their circumstances, then what you've given them is wasted. So, that's what our foundation is all about. It's about teaching people how to fish.

Wright

So, do you work with them one-on-one?

Blanks

We can do both; we have an opportunity to work with them one-on-one, and then we also have the opportunity to actually go there and see the program our foundation is donating to. If their cause is what we want to donate to, then we don't really have to work with them because the program is doing what we think is needed for the public.

Wright

You stated, in one of the things I read, that the Billy Blanks foundation focuses on the "ripple effect." What do you mean by that?

Blanks

Well, you throw a rock in a pond, and it causes things to happen. I believe when you take a young kid and teach him something it causes a ripple effect. If a kid learns something it goes to his brain and starts to register. The kid thinks, "Well you know, if I can be successful here, then I can be successful in other things in my life." That's why we call it the ripple effect. You cause a reaction, and the reaction causes you to go on to become successful at other things.

Wright

Well, it's sure working out with you. Isn't your daughter working in your Karate studio with you?

Blanks

Yes. My daughter travels with me all over the world, and I think it's truly a blessing to be able to have her doing things along with her father; to go out there and teach a class and speak to people about how to get their life together. I think it's awesome. You know, it's doing the right thing in the eyes of your kids and in the hearts of your kids—showing them that in order to be the best you can be, it takes work, it takes belief, and it takes loving—loving yourself and loving people.

Wright

I read that while you were training in your home, you began to combine dance movements with Tae Kwon Do, which evolved into TaeBo. Is that right? Were you the originator of TaeBo?

Blanks

Yes, you know what happened? My wife went out and bought the *Rocky* theme song.

Wright

Oh, yes.

Blanks

When you put that song on, it just makes you want to move. I had just won the United States championship, and after I won it, I went downstairs in the basement and put on the album. I started moving to the music. The song was probably no more than three or four minutes long, and within that period of time, I got tired. It was a real cardiovascular workout. I thought, "Wow! This is bad for *me* to be getting tired." What I started doing then was to add Karate movements to the music. I started seeing my cardiovascular system increase in efficiency. Most martial arts guys don't have workouts that include cardiovascular exercises—they only use Karate techniques.

Wright

I understand.

Blanks

So, I started adding Karate movements to music and adding boxing movements. Then I began adding calisthenics. When I put it all together I had created a system for myself to get in good shape. When my wife came down to the basement and saw what I was doing, she said, "Billy, you should teach this to women." So, I ended up teaching her for a couple of weeks, and she saw a difference. Her body started to change, and her attitude started to change by working out.

I went to a hair salon and asked women there if I could give them TaeBo classes, and they said sure. I gave them one class, and after class they asked if I could do it two days a week. That's how TaeBo started to kick in. I then ended up moving to California and met Paula Abdul. I talked to her about the class and started teaching her and Catherine Bach (the lady who played Daisy Duke on the television series "Dukes of Hazzard").

Wright

Of course.

Blanks

Well, I started training her, and then I introduced them to TaeBo. The next thing you know, well, it just started to take off.

Wright

All of my friends have your tapes. And, as a matter of fact, one of the ladies who works in the office knew I was going to talk with you today and told me she thought you were the greatest thing in the world! I guess the dance is what makes it interesting. I tried running for a long time, and I have never seen anybody run with a smile on his or her face. Dancing must be a little bit different. Is that why it's so popular?

Blanks

No, you know what it is? I believe that the reason TaeBo has touched the world is because it touches the heart of a person; it tells them the truth about physical fitness. It doesn't lie to them. I didn't say people would get in shape easily. I told them, "If you have a will, there's a way for you to get in shape, but it's going to take hard work, it's going to take effort, it's going to take everything you have to push yourself to be the best that you can be." People heard what I was saying, and they went out and tried it. They saw it was a challenge—not to the body, it was a challenge to the will—to be able to make it through that class. As they started to see that it was a challenge, this made them accept it. After they started to get involved with learning how to do TaeBo, then it became not just an exercise, it became a workout that taught how to communicate with your body. People started to learn what their body could do and what it couldn't do. And, the next thing you know, they started thinking, "My kicks are getting higher, my balance is getting better, and my flexibility is getting better." It was developing them from the inside out instead of the outside in.

I believe people started to train themselves on being able to kick faster, kick higher, have more flexibility, punch harder, and move to the music instead of concentrating only on what they looked like. So, TaeBo combined other elements that made them become blind to what they were seeing in the mirror. Eventually, six or seven months later, when they did look in the mirror, they saw their body had lost inches and size. I think that's why TaeBo is out there right now—it's giving people a chance to make physical fitness become a lifestyle more than just an exercise regimen—a trend that people usually work on for six months and then give up.

Wright

How often do you suggest doing it?

Blanks

I always tell people to start off with two or three times a week. Even if you have only ten minutes out of a day, take that time and help yourself learn how to educate your body and how to communicate with your body so that you understand how to get yourself in good shape.

Most people don't work out. They don't really know what their body can do. It's like my being on the telephone with you, what I'm doing is communicating, and you're giving me the opportunity to communicate with millions of people. The same thing is true with TaeBo. TaeBo gives you the chance to communicate with your body, it gives you the chance to understand what your legs and arms can be used for—other than walking and picking up things—what your mind can do, what your will can do, and how far you can push yourself. There's so much to be learned about yourself when you're out there exercising that will help you in everyday life.

Wright

You used the three words there that are synonymous with mind, body, and spirit. Is that what it's about?

Blanks

That's what I call it: mind, soul, and, body.

Wright

You know, at the expense of sounding like a namedropper, I was impressed with some of your clientele—Paula Abdul, Rebecca De Mornay, Connie Selleca, Ryan O'Neal, Sinbad, Magic Johnson, Shaquille O'Neal, Bruce Jenner—I know, I'm cutting the list really short. Because of their jobs and their image, these people have to look good and feel good. How did you ever attract such a group of celebrities?

Blanks

Well, I think the celebrities came by hearing about it from everyday people who were saying, "Hey, man, you should go down and try this class out. This is where I'm working out, and this guy pushes you." This studio is built on not just celebrities, but it's built on everyday people. Everyday people come in here, and want to work out—they all want to get in shape. They go out and they talk to people. People start to talk to people who know people, and, the next thing you know, celebrities are in the class because of someone out there at home or a mother or a daughter who has spoken to maybe a father, and the father might be an agent. So, it's just communication skills, them going around telling another person, "You know, if you want to get into good shape, go to Billy Blanks; he'll really push you to the limit."

A lot of the athletes, actors and singers come down here to work out, and they're all treated just like regular people, they all get in line like regular people. I don't charge them any differently; they all pay the same price. Everybody wants to get in shape; it doesn't matter if he or she is a celebrity, or an everyday person. All these people have the same desire; they all want to be the best they can be. So, that's the way I look at it. I view it as a blessing to have them all in the studio, to have them all in here all together, doing the same thing—exercising their will and getting themselves in the best shape they can get in.

Wright

Billy, we're trying to encourage people in our audience to be better, to live better, and be more fulfilled by listening to the examples of our guests. Is there anything or anyone in your life who has really made a difference to you and helped you become a better person?

Blanks

Yes, I would say one gentleman, Pastor Price—Fredrick Casey Price. He actually turned my whole life around.

Wright

How did he do it?

Blanks

Well, when I saw him on television preaching the Gospel, it gave me a better understanding of who Jesus Christ is. When I accepted Jesus Christ in my life, it was a big turn for me. I didn't have to be searching for what the world had to offer me anymore; I had to search for what God had to offer me. It was fulfilling to know that having Him in my life had made a big change. Being around a man who really loves God, who is not compromising about God's Word, who walks his talk, gives me the opportunity to see that a regular man can be like God said he could be. And, that's awesome to me.

Wright

How old were you?

Blanks

I was actually, let's see, it was six and a half years ago.

Wright

So, was Gayle a Christian before that?

Blanks

No, actually, the same thing happened to her. I was the first person who went to church. I was always trying to get her to go to the church, and she wouldn't go. She had had some bad experiences. I asked her to, "Just listen to the man." And one day, he was talking on the television about faith. All of a sudden I looked behind me and saw her there. I told her, "Here's the guy I was telling you about, listen to him on TV." She actually took the covers and pulled them over her head. She didn't want to listen. Then he said something about faith. When I looked back I saw the covers started coming off her head, she sat up, and started watching TV. Eventually, she asked me to take her to the church, so, I took her to church and that day, she received Jesus Christ. And now we all go to church, including my daughter. It is truly a blessing to be able to have Jesus Christ in your life, giving you so many more opportunities to be the best that you can be.

Wright

What do you think makes a great mentor? In other words, are there characteristics mentors seem to have in common?

Blanks

Yes. I think what makes up a good mentor is a person who has good beliefs; he's not a compromising person; he stands on his word.

Wright

You've certainly been a mentor for a lot of young people, especially since you treat everybody the same, don't you?

Blanks

Yes, I treat everybody the same. We all are people, we all want to be loved, and we all want to be careful, you know? I want to help someone as much as they want to be helped. That's why I love Jesus Christ, that's why every time I do something, I want people to see Jesus in me. That's what He was all about. His goal was to seek and to save, and that's what I'm all about, and that's what my daughter's all about; the same goes for my wife and the people who are around me. Our goal is to seek and save and help as many people as we can help while here on earth.

Wright

I was reading some of your movie and television credits. I couldn't believe it. You've been in some great sitcoms: "Suddenly Susan," "Spencer for Hire," "Melrose Place," "Hard Copy." Is that something you really enjoy doing?

Blanks

Yes, it's fun. It's been a blessing to be able to go out there and be on TV and win a Karate championship and do the things I've been doing. Who would ever have thought I would be doing that? I thought of it, I had belief that I would do it. To actually be able to be there and give credit to God is an awesome thing. I always say God is the Creator who gives us the opportunity to be the best we can be. For me to be able to be on television, do a video, and touch so many lives, is truly a blessing.

Wright

Billy, what did faith mean to you up until about six and a half years ago?

Blanks

I didn't really know what faith was until I got involved with Pastor Price and had a chance to understand. I believed I could be a champion, but I didn't know that was a big part of faith. I didn't know that man had natural faith until I opened up the Bible and started learning about it. It was awesome to me to know that I was establishing my life as a young man on unseen evidence, believing that I could obtain that goal by hard work. Then, as I got involved in the Word of God, all of a sudden I got a chance to review and see how I got to where I am. Now I know how to become a better person. I ask myself, "Well, what if I could have had faith in God in my life when I was growing up and had had the understanding then that I have right now? How much better would I be?" Obviously, you can't go backwards so I always say, "Well, I just thank God for where I am today, because that's why I am here." It's because I got the opportunity to acknowledge what God can do for me as an older adult. I always tell people out there, "You know, there's nothing better than being able to know something about faith and understanding God's Word."

Wright

Well, Someone must have been looking out for you. Gayle was your high school sweetheart, wasn't she?

Blanks

Yes, I always say, "My wife is my spinal cord." Without my spinal cord, I can't walk around right? We've been married for twenty-eight years now, and it's truly a blessing to be able to have somebody who can deal with an athlete. Athletes, sometimes, are hard people to deal with, and my wife has put up with me for a long time, so I take my hat off to her. Without her as my spinal cord, I would never be where I am today.

Wright

I was talking with Les Brown the other day; he's a motivational speaker and a fine man. Les told me just about the same story I read about you. As a child his inattention to schoolwork, his restless energy, and the failure of his teachers to recognize his true potential resulted in him being mislabeled as a slow learner. He thought he was a loser, and stupid, and dumb, but now he's one of the world's leading motivational speakers

Blanks

That is so awesome.

Wright

How was your dyslexia diagnosed?

Blanks

You know what happened? My wife and I were sitting in a parking lot, and we were reading this sign, it was a Karate sign on a Karate studio building. I looked up and saw this sign and I read it backwards. Then she read it and we got into an argument about who was reading it right. She finally said, "Billy, you're reading that sign wrong," and I said, "No *you're* reading it wrong; you look at it." She looked at it, and I looked at it, and I said, "You read it." So she read it, and then she asked me to read it, and I read it. Then I saw I was reading it backwards. Then we went to a clinic that helped dyslexic people and it was there I was diagnosed as being a dyslexic.

Wright

I bet that was life changing wasn't it?

Blanks

You know, it *was* life changing, but what happened to me was that it really gave me a sense of understanding. I thank God for being able to have that, because who would ever think I would be where I am today? I mean, I've made it to being the world champion, I made it to being one of the best trainers in the business, I've made it to being able to talk to people, and I was written off as retarded and stupid. So, to be able to achieve those goals, knowing I was dyslexic enhanced my abilities to want to go on and say, "Wow! If I had known this when I was younger, how much better could I have become?"

Even though I've had to learn in a different way to become just as wise as other young people, I thank God for being able to acknowledge that even though I am dyslexic, I still became successful in life by hard work and acquiring understanding about how to achieve my goals through other means. As I was taken through testing and given activities to help me become better, I became stronger and gained confidence about everything else that I do.

To tell kids and others about being dyslexic wasn't hard for me to do because I think it was a good testimony. Some young person might be sitting in my audience and they might need somebody to say, "Well, I'm dyslexic and look where I am because I put God first, and I thank God for what I do, through hard work and believing that I can overcome. Look at where I stand now." I'm going all over the world speaking to people hoping to help anyone who might need to hear this.

Wright

My wife does the same thing. She's a cancer survivor and uses her experience to motivate people. She says, "If I can do it, you can do it!" It's easy to understand why you're a great mentor to young people.

Blanks

Well, thank you.

Wright

Most people are fascinated right now with all these new reality television shows about being a survivor. What has been the greatest comeback from adversity you have ever made? Was it the fact that you were disadvantaged when you were younger or something else?

Blanks

Well, in my adult life, I had my knee operated on because it became separated. It bent backward just as far as it did the way that it should bend naturally. I was told I'd never be able to walk again. I didn't accept that because of other parts in my life I believed I could overcome and did overcome. I just kept believing and one day I was able to get my leg back into position and was able to overcome that problem. I am so be blessed to be doing what I'm doing—I can kick, I can punch, and I can run, and that just causes me to say, "See, God is good, God is always like He says He is."

Wright

If you could have a platform and tell our audience something you believe would help them or encourage them, what would you say?

Blanks

I would tell them to walk by faith and not by sight. I continue to say that to everybody around the world. I say that if you can walk by faith and not by sight, you will always make it to where you want to go. Using Jesus Christ as the light, you can make it to where you need to go. He'll give you the power, and He'll give you the strength.

Wright

That's great advice. I really appreciate you being on the program today. It's meant a lot to me. You're an inspiration!

Blanks

Thank you.

Wright

Today we have been talking to Billy Blanks, one of the most sought-after trainers and fitness consultants in the entire world. He has won every kind of championship imaginable. As you can see, that's no surprise. He's also a great, great man. Thank you so much Billy.

About The Author

Billy Blanks

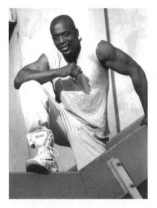

Billy Blanks is the creator of Tae Bo®, the revolutionary total body fitness system that has helped millions of people around the world get in shape and feel great! He has also devoted a great deal of time toward helping people through his Foundation and by traveling around the world to train the U.S. Armed Forces. In addition, Billy has made extraordinary achievements as a world karate champion, actor, author, motivator, philanthropist and humanitarian. Billy's rise to success seems all the more astonishing when seen through the prism of his childhood. Born the fourth of fifteen children to Isaac and Mabeline Blanks, he had few opportunities on the mean streets of Erie, Pennsylvania. Complicating his young life, Billy was afflicted with undiagnosed dyslexia and suffered a problem in his hip joints, which impaired his movement, resulting in a clumsiness that caused his coaches to think he would never amount to much. Billy moved to Boston as an adult and opened his own karate studio. It was there that while combining dance moves and Tae Kwon Do, he unintentionally hit upon the concept for Tae Bo®. Blanks then moved to Los Angeles in 1989 and taught classes in his garage. Shortly after, he opened the Billy Blanks World Training Center in Sherman Oaks.

Billy Blanks
www.billyblanks.com

Chapter 13

Good Humor Is Good Medicine

Johnny Burns, MHA, CHE

How do you feel after a good hearty laugh? Does it leave you depressed or uplifted? Does it leave you energized or exhausted? Does it feel good or does it feel bad? As a healthcare executive for the past twenty years and a part-time comedian/humorist for the last few years, I have learned unequivocally that "Good Humor is Good Medicine."

Just these two job positions in juxtaposition—healthcare executive and part-time comedian—have to be considered incongruously humorous by some. What can possibly be funny about being sick, or about healthcare for that matter? The answer is—everything—if you let it.

A couple of years ago I had a colonoscopy, a procedure not usually considered fun (well, maybe by some, but not by most of us). The greatest and the worst thing about being a humorist is that you are expected to find humor in just about everything. So, following the embarrassment of this procedure, I found the humor in the encounter. I did this by crafting a speech, which, amazingly enough, has become one of my most requested: "My Colonoscopy. Why it Pays Not to Get in Arrears with Your Proctologist."

Now, why would I do such a thing? Is the first thing that goes through a person's mind when they are having a colonoscopy, "Hey, I should write this down in detail and tell the world about it. They'll want to know"? Probably not, unless the person is a sa-

221

dist, a masochist, a doctor...or a humorist. I'm one of those. Healthcare is serious business, which is why it needs a humorist—just as life is serious business, which is why it needs *lots* of humorists. This is why jokes and joking around exist—they take the edge off the chronic seriousness of life. We all need to become part-time humorists—people who specialize in or who are noted for humor, at least part of the time. Wouldn't you like to be someone noted for good humor? Would that appall you or appeal to you? I bet the latter. Good humor is not just about getting laughs or telling jokes—it's deeper inside. It's an attitude that life can be fun and rewarding—that successful doesn't have to mean stressful.

There's a seminar I give to middle level managers called "The Monkeys of Management: How to Keep Them off Your Back!" The seminar addresses key issues that managers and supervisors face in any business operation. This includes topics such as people management, financial management, marketing, customer service, and time- and self-organization. When I start this seminar, stuffed monkeys are all over my back and hanging around my shoulders and clasped to my legs. It always gets a laugh when I enter to the sound of monkeys squeaking and squealing. Why? It's because folks understand the stresses and pressures of having these "monkeys" on their backs. They appreciate it being presented in a light and humorous vein. Their problems are real, they feel the monkeys are real, and they welcome the comic relief. The seminar gives practical approaches and solutions to managing their monkeys, but it does so in a humorous, fun, and entertaining way—something they (the managers, not the monkeys) are not accustomed to experiencing in their work place.

Humor breaks up negative thought patterns. It opens the receiver up to new ways to address problems, and it lets folks know that it is okay to laugh. Viktor Fankl, in his book, *Man's Search for Meaning*, states that some of the prisoners of war in Hitler's concentration camps chose to use humor to relieve the stress and pressures of their incomprehensible life in these Nazi compounds. Certain groups would cope with the pressure by setting aside time to meet—frequently meaning they might have to forgo a meager meal—just to share jokes and funny experiences. This gave them some solace in conditions that were barbarian. He attributes these sessions for giving hope to many who were incarcerated there. Frankl wrote, "I would never have made it if I could not have laughed. Laughing lifted me momentarily . . . out of this horrible situation, just enough to make it livable . . . survivable."

If even in the conditions experienced by prisoners of war people can find and use humor to get them through, don't you think we can too? Humor helps restore life's balance and creates perspective. You rarely hear anyone say, "I've been laughing so much lately I feel depressed." If you do, avoid those people. They probably are members of S.A. (Serious Anonymous) or they are consuming vast quantities of non-prescription drugs. Alternatively it could mean they have been spending so much time in comedy clubs they've lost their jobs.

There is nothing depressing about laughter...well, unless the people who are laughing are pointing at you derisively because your zipper is down in the middle of your wedding. No, that did not happen to me, I don't care what you heard!

In the healthcare field there are a lot of analysts. There are scientific analysts. There are physician analysts. In some circles they are called proctologists (that's an inside joke). There are financial analysts. There are even pieces of laboratory equipment called analyzers. So it would seem to be appropriate to medically dissect and analyze humor; however we won't do that here. It seems counter-productive to over-analyze laughter. Heck, we all know laughter is good for us, except for maybe, librarians and state troopers.

Scientifically, laughter increases many of our natural killer cells. These "killer" cells are the type that fight and often destroy tumors and viruses. With laughter there is also an increase of T-cells essential for our immune system, and B-cells which generate antibodies that fight disease. And, if that is not enough to have you channel surfing for a sit-com or an extreme humor makeover, laughter also causes an elevation (and this is quite scientific so stick with me here) of Gamma-interferon—the body's disease fighting protein. Now, lest you were wondering, Gamma-interferon is *not* a substance currently banned by major league baseball.

Shakespeare wrote, "Nothing is good or bad. It is thinking that makes it so." The next time you say quietly to yourself, or even out loud, if prone to outbursts, "I think it's going to be a bad day," guess what? It's *going* to be a bad day, not because Shakespeare said so (he didn't even know you) but because *you* said so. So you influence your health by your attitude. Starting each day with a good attitude is a good start to becoming a good humor person. (No, you don't have to sell ice cream.) To paraphrase Shakespeare: think good—feel good.

In high school, my son Adam performed in the great classic play *Oklahoma*. He was the comic character, peddler Ali Hakim. (What can I say, humor runs in the family.) But in that play there is a great song that goes something like this, "Oh what a beautiful morning, oh what a beautiful day. I've got a beautiful feeling everything's going my way." Isn't that exquisite, even if it was a semi-western? I sing those lines to myself (be warned my singing voice is not for public consumption) on mornings and other times when I start to have negative thoughts. It mostly works and leaves me in a good humor. Try it. You'll like it. Remember Shakespeare, "It is thinking that makes it so."

Did you ever notice that kids seem to have a lot more fun than adults do? Does an increase in knowledge over the years cause chronic seriousness? Apparently so. Kids of nursery school age laugh about 300 times a day, and adults average only about seventeen laughs a day. Darn. This is not a good thing. We need to humor up. It may be good for us to lower our cholesterol score but it is not good to lower our laugh score. Raise it, now. So if you want to stay healthy, have an apple and 300 laughs a day. That's far more manageable than a laugh and 300 apples a day. This brings to mind a quote from Voltaire (no, I did not hear this from him personally). He said, "The art of medicine consists of keeping the patient amused while nature heals the disease." Across the ages it appears true that good humor is good medicine.

Remember the time in school, or at church, or in a workplace meeting when you got the giggles and just couldn't stifle the laugh? You knew that it wasn't acceptable but your body wanted to, needed to, and intended to laugh. Even through your embarrassment you knew it felt good, even if inappropriate at the time. It felt so good to laugh you just had to do it. Then there were those times, even among the most serious of us (yes, even a humorist has a serious side, for me it's my left side) got caught up with someone else's giggling or laughing fit. Soon everybody was tickled to death. It was more contagious than the Macarena.

Why do we say that—"tickled to death"? I have visited all but a couple of the states in the U.S.A. and over a dozen foreign countries. I have yet to see or hear of anyone who has laughed

themselves to death or who has passed away due to others tick-
ling them. On the other hand there's the saying, "I laughed so
hard I wet my pants." Now you don't have to travel too far to find
someone who has done that (my sister Debbie comes to mind).
Maybe that's why kids laugh more than we do—they are accustomed to wetting their pants—no big deal. Certainly it is no
reason to stop laughing.

Now if any of you are saying, regarding the pants-wetting
thing, that I have just given you a good reason not to laugh, forget
it. No, what I have given you is a good reason to consider adding
adult diapers to your wardrobe, which, as of yet, do not come in
designer colors. Whether or not you need them "depends" on the
quality, the length, and the complexity of the laugh; besides,
there are meds for that—it's all scientific.

When I say that humor is good medicine I am not saying that
it cures any specific disease, but I am confident that it helps.
Maybe it is prophylactic. Maybe it is palliative. Maybe it is psychiatric. It certainly puts the body in a better position to defend
itself against disease and stave off the ill effects, physical and
psychological, of stress. In his book, *The Anatomy of an Illness,*
Norman Cousins, former editor of *Saturday Review,* credits
laughter for helping him recover from a potentially fatal disease.

Consider some of the positive effects laughter can have on your
body, your mind, and your spirit. It helps reduce stress and lower
your blood pressure. It elevates your mood and provides a natural
boost to your immune system. It improves brain functioning and
helps to protect your heart. Wow! Johnny, if laughter can do that
for me, bring it on! But wait—there's more.

Sure, laughter can help improve your mind, your body, and
your spirit, but it can also aid you socially and professionally.
How can that be? Think about it. Who are people drawn to?
They're drawn to someone who makes them feel comfortable.
People are attracted to folks with a good sense of humor, not to
the curmudgeons, crabs, and creeps. A sense of humor, a smile,
and a shared laugh connects you with others. It can help foster
relationships and create relaxation. In general, good humor is a
valued attribute in our friends, our family, and our co-workers.
Good humor makes for good feelings, and when you feel good, life
gets better.

As much as laughter and good humor helps the living, it also
has a profound effect on the dying. There are countless stories

shared by hospice nurses of how a positive sense of humor has helped the process of dying for terminally ill patients and their families. I will share one such story with you. It is one that is poignantly personal. It is about a hospice patient with paternal connections—my father.

Before continuing, let me digress a bit and tell you a few facts about my dad, the once indefatigable J. J. Burns. He was a Georgia farm boy with a great sense of humor. People were drawn to him because he was fun to be around. He made people feel good. He really liked and cared about people and it showed. He enlisted in the Army at an early age and served in France during World War II, which possibly explained his love of cheese, red wine, and the phrase "c'est la vie."

Now, not only did Dad love people, he loved life and lived it fully. By "living it fully" I mean he worked hard, he played hard, and he had lots of fun. Sometimes he had too much fun and occasionally got into a little trouble, especially with my mom; but he always bounced back with his great sense of humor and great sense of life. With over thirty years of service in the military, he retired a Command Sergeant Major after experiencing a near fatal massive heart attack at the age of forty-nine. This occurred while he was chopping down a tree for my Fat Granny. Whoa! Did I just say "Fat Granny?" Isn't that rude—maybe even politically incorrect? Well perhaps these days, yes, but I had two grandmothers growing up. One was Little Granny and the other was Fat Granny and that's how we referred to them our whole lives, even after my sisters, my brother, and I grew up. It was never said with disrespect, and Fat Granny actually liked it. She was a woman who had a great sense of humor and wow! Could she ever cook and eat! She was a large, good-humored woman who made the best chicken and dumplings and biscuits in the world.

So, while cutting down this tree in Fat Granny's garden, my father experienced crushing chest pains. At the hospital they said he was not expected to live, so I traveled from New Orleans where I was attending Tulane University to be with him. In the hospital I found my father hooked up to tubes, lines, wires, oxygen, etcetera, etcetera, etcetera. As was his custom he was always thinking of others first. He tried cheering *me* up by joking around. He said he really didn't care much what those doctors thought because he didn't think it was his time to die. And he did not die. Instead he spent his weeks of recovery in the hospital making the nurses and doctors laugh. When he was discharged to home the hospital staff couldn't comment enough on his positive spirit and good humor. They said he made their jobs easier with his attitude.

In 1969, when they sent him home, they thought he was going home to die. He knew he was going home to live. You have got to love that spirit. Dad was in and out of hospitals many times over the next thirty years. He was always the favorite patient of the nurses and aides because he never griped, he was not demanding, and he made them laugh. How well do you think they took care of him? Very well, thank you. Having a good sense of humor pays dividends in many ways.

Things were much different when his doctor sent him home in 2003. The doctor and Dad both now knew he was going home to die. He was ready and it was okay. His time had come. Before leaving he thanked the nurses, the doctors, and the staff who had cared for him, gave me his final instructions, and headed for home in an ambulance. Of course he kidded and joked with the emergency medical technicians all the way home.

Once home, his only concern seemed to be that family and friends who were there were appropriately entertained. As he sat in his favorite chair, while he was still able to, he received many of his friends who stopped by and he enjoyed visiting with his family. During this time while he was dying he joked and kidded with caretakers, friends, and family. I recall the day one of his sergeant major friends came by to pay his respects. Here are two old soldiers, veterans of World War II, talking about the good and the bad times—times they had fought, the meals they had shared, and times they had played pool in the NCO clubs.

Upon leaving, my father's friend turned to him and said, "J.J., when you get to heaven I want you to save me a place at the table."

My father, two days from death, looked at him said, "dinner or pool?" Humor helps. Make a point to keep humor in your life, regardless of the circumstances.

Whenever I recall my father's last days on earth, I get a little teary. Alright then, I get a lot teary. Well, actually it's more like a tsunami. What can I say? I loved the man. He taught me so much: how to fish, how to wish, and how to live by the golden rule. Most of all he taught me about the power of a positive attitude and a good sense of humor. For my dad, good humor was good medicine. For all of us, good humor is good medicine.

So when my offspring, Adam, decided to drop out of the University of Texas to pursue his dream of acting, writing, and directing, I definitely needed a positive attitude and a good sense of humor. I cannot tell a lie. (Well, I *can*, but I'm not going to right now.) I was not deliriously happy when Adam shared with me his plans to move to Hollywood; but I *was* concerned—concerned, in this instance, meant devastated. I wondered how could a guy who gets a perfect score on the verbal SAT not want to stay in school, especially when I was paying all the bills? I could have ranted, raved, turned red in the face, and made both of our lives miserable. Instead, drawing on all that I teach and preach to others, I urged him to consider the long-term effects on his life and his career. I reminded him that there are some actors who actually got a college degree first. I reminded him that I had saved enough money for him to attend college for four years. I reminded him that I used to be taller than he was. I reminded him of how crestfallen his lovely mother would be. He reminded me that he had, after careful deliberation, made up his mind; at which point all remaining reminders had reached their expiration date.

What could have caused such a bright boy to do such a thing? His mother, my darling wife Cher of thirty plus years, reminded me it was my fault. She did, however, say it in a nice way. (She's a very nice person.) Yes, she reminded me that it was my fault for taking time out from running hospitals to do stand-up comedy and subsequently performing with Adam at the Laugh Stop. We were the first ever father-and-son comedy team to appear at the Laugh Stop in Houston's Funniest Person Contest—twice. Comforted in knowing it was "my fault," Adam headed to Hollywood, where he currently resides.

By now, after sifting through my parenting challenges, you are probably asking yourself, why did Johnny, a hospital administrator, decide to do stand-up comedy? If you weren't asking yourself that question, then you should have been—it's important. Hospital administrators, as a rule, do not do stand-up (comedy, that is). But you see, I wanted even more good humor in my life, so I took a comedy writing course while I was a healthcare CEO. I was giving a lot of local presentations and wanted to "liven them up a bit."

It went well. Based on the monologue I wrote during the class I was asked to perform at a local comedy club. It was a terrifying experience. So I went back and did it again and again. (Go figure.) It even inspired me to create the first humor therapy program in a psychiatric and substance abuse hospital in Houston. I set up a humor room with weird things like presidential blow-up dolls, wooden aquariums, fun house mirrors, and tons of funny audio and videotapes. There were Jeff Foxworthy calendars and jokes of the day, Three Stooges, and Laurel and Hardy films. The patients loved it. The staff thought I was nuts, and then they loved it (job security). The media loved it. The owners of the hospital gave me an award. (It was cheaper than giving me a raise.) Good humor is wonderful. Try it—you'll like it.

I recently learned of a radiation oncology practice that goes the extra mile to create an environment of good humor and positive feelings for its patients undergoing treatment for cancer. They put smiley faces all over the center and only hire friendly, smiling staff members (this is not a governmental facility). They make the patients feel that everybody there considers them their friend. One of the doctors there was recently recognized as a "Super Doc" in Texas because of his total commitment to helping his patients, not only medically, but psychologically as well.

I read some of his patients' anonymous comments on feedback forms. The comments were fabulous. Most CEOs in America would give up partial stock options for these kinds of satisfied customers. Here is an example, "The humor and frivolity reduced the stress of the threat of cancer." How about that? Once again, good humor is good medicine. And good business.

This doctor and his practice are much more attuned to what their patients want and need than most businesses are. Sure, they would all like to be cured of cancer. They would also like the treatment and the treatment team to have human qualities. They would like to be in good humor during the treatment, if at all possible. If you were being treated for cancer would you rather be treated scientifically, efficiently, and medically with no regard to your psyche? Or would you want the treatment to be sprinkled with good times, good humor, a few laughs, and folks who know, understand, and practice a good positive attitude? I know my answer.

Yet there are doctors, lawyers, and many other professionals who look upon their clients as an intrusion into their lives. Imagine the doctor who says, "My patients are so sick and needy. It's really draining me." Wait just a medical minute here, doctor. If they weren't sick, would they need you? If they didn't need you would you be able to "practice" all that cool stuff you learned in medical school and during the process be able to pay back the gazillion dollars you owe in medical school loans?

Many people believe it is easier to have a good sense of humor if you don't have much pressure in your life. Excuse me here, but they are wrong. Frequently it is the "pressure" that gives us the basis for humor. I served as a military officer—U.S. Army—during the wind down of the Vietnam War. I was trained as an infantry officer, I was a parachutist, I completed rotary wing basic and advanced flight school, and became a helicopter test pilot for the 82nd Airborne Division at Fort Bragg. Had I not had a sense of humor I would never have survived that stuff: learning to use lethal weapons, putting up with drill sergeants, sleeping in large tents with little or no privacy, taking the first solo flight without an instructor pilot, jumping out of an airplane that was at least half a mile high, and eating food that defied description in Army mess halls. I wouldn't trade those pressures for anything, or the humor that could be found in all of them.

These life events were both fun and entertaining to me, albeit, at times, quite stressful, but mostly because I used humor to lighten the load. While in flight school, a good friend and I became the entertainment for our fellow classmates, the Green Hats. (Each class was named according to the color of the baseball caps assigned to their class. If you were wondering, ours was green.) So Gary and I became song masters. Gary could sing, I could write (which has become less evident as I have aged). So, like Rodgers and Hammerstein, we composed crazy lyrics to fit our circumstances. Our fellow classmates and the instructors loved it—the fact that we were willing to make fools of ourselves and risk our status as commissioned officers all in the name of fun. But the humor pulled us through; it reduced the stress and it relieved the tension. I'd share one of our songs but it wouldn't make much sense if you hadn't been there. But if you had been there—oh yeah, we had fun; especially as we progressed through the course to the point that our instructors no longer considered us aviation morons and flying klutzes. The Green Hats became legend...at least in our own minds.

A positive sense of humor is not only medicine for your body and mind, it is a tonic for your soul. Fellow NSA members, Jack Canfield and Mark Victor Hansen, wrote a wonderful book called

Chicken Soup for the Soul. I believe that the right attitude and a positive sense of humor can create "Good Humor Bars for the Soul." It doesn't sound as pretty but it works just as well. By lifting your spirits and those around you, humor lightens life's burdens and brightens the future. It makes life sweeter.

Humor also can also endear you to your spouse. If there's one thing my wife and I have done right, it is to communicate. We talk a lot, sometimes to each other, mostly to the dog. (Just kidding. The dog doesn't talk, but she is a great listener). I say a lot of dumb things. My wife laughs at them, or maybe at me. It doesn't matter. But we connect with humor.

While I was out of town on one of my many business trips not long ago, she sent me an e-mail. The e-mail was only seven words, and it lifts my spirits to this day. It read, "You are fun and exciting and brilliant." Just as my ego was soaring I decided it was actually one of those spam things, so I double-checked; but lo and behold she had actually addressed it to *me*. I was elated, on cloud nine, even ebullient (although I have no idea what that word means). I was suddenly a fun and exciting and brilliant man! It was one person's opinion and, surprisingly enough, I shared it.

Evidently good humor is not only good for your health but also your marriage. It doesn't hurt with raising kids either. My daughter Emily, who did *not* drop out of the University of Texas, laughs at me all the time. She thinks I'm funny, or was the word goofy? I forget. Emily's sense of humor is bit more subtle than mine, but she is witty and pretty and bright. I am guessing her sense of humor will continue to benefit her in life.

When Adam and Emily were younger, I learned to juggle to entertain them and their friends. I would dress up strangely (fish net stockings were not part of the scene) and juggle and act like an idiot (maybe I wasn't acting), and they would laugh. I would make up stories and let them all choose characters or items that I would weave into the stories. One of the recurrent scenarios involved me performing part of the story in a closet and then emerging from the closet in character with much fanfare. The kids loved this. Although it nearly caused problems when Emily told her friends' parents that her dad was coming out of the closet. I almost got banned from the guys' Friday night poker games.

Good humor definitely is good medicine if it helps with child rearing and spousal relations. We all know that stress is a major contributor to illness. Anything that helps reduce that stress is useful in preventing some types of illness. Well, not *anything*. If you use drugs or booze to relieve your stress it may backfire on you; but humor is a good way of reducing this stress. The label on the good humor bottle says there are no ill side effects. Hey! Even aspirin has side effects. With laughter there are no drug interaction warnings. That just shows how good humor can be for you. The FDA has never recalled laughter. Great. We can all agree that humor makes you feel good, and it reduces stress which in turn staves off illnesses. Isn't it about time you increased your daily dosage of humor? Of course it is. Take time to read the comics. Get a joke-a-day calendar. I love the ones Jeff Foxworthy has. Smile and make others smile. Laugh out loud a lot. Read and watch funny stuff. Practice good humor, and you will be rewarded in many ways.

It has been proven that, over a period of time, people who laugh regularly tend to have lower blood pressure than those who don't. You see, what happens is, when folks have a hearty laugh their blood pressure initially increases but then lowers to below normal levels. When we laugh we breathe deeper and give more oxygen to the blood, and our heart happily sends this enriched blood to the rest of our body. There is nothing wrong with having happy enriched blood coursing through your body.

The Serenity Prayer used in many twelve step programs says "God grant me the serenity to accept the things I cannot change; courage to change the things I can; and wisdom to know the difference." You can change yourself into a good humor person. You can choose to be more positive, upbeat, and fun. Do it now. After all, it is good medicine and it makes life so much more enjoyable. Who knows? One day you may receive an e-mail that tells you that you are fun, exciting, and brilliant.

About The Author

Johnny Burns, MHA, CHE

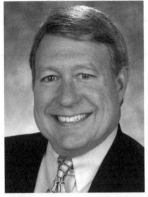

Johnny Burns has a unique set of experiences. He has a Master's Degree in Health Administration; has served as a sales representative, corporate executive, hospital CEO; and was an officer, paratrooper, and helicopter test pilot for the US Army. He is an entrepreneur, a consultant, a trainer, and has appeared in comedy clubs including the Laff Stop and The Improv. His take on life, relationships, health matters, leadership and communications is entertaining, educational and enlightening - laughter with a message! Johnny has presented to various trade associations, healthcare organizations, Fortune 500 corporations, hospitals, civic groups, governmental entities and the military. Skillfully using humor, he provides keynotes, breakouts, roasts, seminars, and other similar presentations regarding all things health, healthcare, and life, as well as business related topics such as mental health, personal growth, stress, success, and customer satisfaction.

Johnny Burns, MHA, CHE
America's Healthcare Humorist
14537 Misty Meadow Lane
Houston, Texas 77079
www.healthhumorist.com
Phone: 713.882.4432
Email: healthhumorist@aol.com

Chapter 14

HOLY SMOKES
AKA How I lost my best friend Cigẽ and found a new light...

Pat McGill

Some thoughts...

I think smokers are selfish, and we are also too easy of a target. We are slaves to a filthy habit. We cough, we pollute the air, we set bad examples for kids, and we know we are harming our health, but we smoke anyway.

We are unlike alcoholics and drug addicts because we can't even call our lack of self-control an illness.

Smokers are losers—or so many non-smokers think. Many of us smokers started before the health risks were known and can't quit now. There were days in my life when I would go without food and buy my cigarettes.

Cigarettes have been a major part of our cultural history. We all know about cigarettes and their use during wartime, about their place in the soldier's life and their use as a tool to manage anxiety, particularly in the face of death. Smokers have been media stars, too. Cigarettes have filled movie screens. Remember that most cinematic smoke, the Humphrey Bogart cigarette? (Tobacco companies are still hooking young smokers with the subtle messages in movies and other media about how "cool" smoking is even though they claim to be doing the opposite.) The fact that there is any march against cigarettes at *all* in this country is ironic when one considers that the government still subsidizes tobacco and encourages its export to other countries.

We need programs to help smokers quit! Smoking may be a blight, but there are ways to address that blight. Public education campaigns, affordable quit smoking programs, and laws restricting smoking in public places are the best ways to attack it.

* Adapted by Pat McGill from "Not Fair to Smokers" by Rekha Basu, *Des Moines Register*, Sunday, February 13, 2005, and *Cigarettes Are Sublime* by Richard Klein.

When I quit smoking (the final time), I began to write *HOLY SMOKES*. I knew smoking was bad for me, and that is why cigarettes were good! Rather a mixed blessing, I'd say now—

We all know it: Tobacco use is the leading single cause of preventable deaths in the United States. Each year tobacco kills more people than traffic accidents, AIDS, alcohol and drug abuse, fire, homicide, and suicide combined. Tobacco causes one out of every five deaths in the United States. Smoking bans and warnings at one time in my life were red flags. Just as I had learned to turn the television channels, every time I heard Yul Brenner warning smokers in his old public service announcements, I was learning to tune out the admonishments from concerned friends. I did not want to hear the ads or the warnings; they made too much sense.

Today I know and understand how important smoking bans are, because they will help encourage smokers to quit their habit, and they improve the health of those who don't smoke. It's that simple: Second hand smoke kills! Thirty seconds of exposure to secondhand smoke increases the stickiness of blood platelets and fosters the formation of plaque inside arteries—plaque that can lead to heart attacks and stroke. Nicotine reaches the brain within seven seconds and can cause problems.

Let's face it, smoking is an emotional issue, and smoke addicts LOVE TO SMOKE! So we need to Start to Stop. The average ex-smoker has started to stop seven times before finally kicking the habit for good. Find that one great reason for *you* to quit; find the passion and purpose to quit smoking, and be prepared to be compassionate to yourself—we are all imperfect human beings with warts.

When I thought about my plan to quit smoking, I started to count the actual cigarettes I had probably smoked off and on over the previous forty years. I stopped counting—it was too depressing. It is tough to think about quitting and tougher to actually quit. Oh, but is it worth it? YES!

For years I thought it couldn't happen to me. Yet, I started to notice health issues, and then the skin cancer alert arrived, and I took notice. I thought, you know, I might just be more attractive at sixty than I was at fifty without my smoker's cough, cigarette breath, and yellowing teeth and fingers. It's not too late at any age to be the best version of yourself! We as smokers must address our physical and psychological addictions for, my dear friends, they are woven together, and I want to tell you to dance with both partners—the physical and the psychological—because you must teach yourself that smoking is a negative, and quitting is the positive.

My Smoking Experiences

I never smoked as a high school student. Instead, I started smoking at the age of nineteen during my first year of college. My smoking was greatly influenced by college itself. Oh, that sounds great—I was away from home at school, and insecurity brought me to "Cigarette Land." No, that wasn't it. I tried a cigarette one night to stay up late and study. The combination of coffee, cigs, and study worked! At the first drag, I knew I liked the taste. My first cigarette created my addiction: *I was a smoker!*

I had quit smoking several times during different periods of time. Really, at times I never thought of myself as "one of those smokers" because I was always going to quit: "I'll quit when this happens; I'll quit when I finish my Master's; when I finish my writing; I promise, then I'll quit." I was not proud of the fact that I was a smoker.

When I took the first drag, I honestly did not know all of the dangers, nor did I know the strength of my new addiction. I share with you in *HOLY SMOKES* my journey to becoming smoke-free. There is not an easy way to quit. *You have to want to quit* and realize that it will be *hell* for a period of time without the drug called nicotine. It's a narcotic. No two ways about it—nicotine is one strong drug, a monkey on your back. No it's more like a Mac truck you are taking everywhere with you because you have to check every place out you go today just on the basis of whether it features a smoking section. Can I smoke there? If not, where I can go to smoke? Does the café have a smoking section? Will the people I am meeting for drinks mind if I smoke? Oh, they do? Really? I guess I'll see you later.

I did go "cold turkey" in a "warm chicken" sort of way. I prepared the process—the plan. This time I was going to quit for good. Forty-six million Americans want to quit smoking, and I was one of them. We all know how much money we spend on cigarettes. I don't have to do the math, and, yes, there were times, when I was younger, when I would go without food and buy cigarettes instead, especially in college. To think I was gaining all that knowledge and doing something that dumb; but I was addicted.

Some Observations...

In Malcolm Gladwell's book *The Tipping Point*, he discusses interesting observations about smoking. I am grateful for his research, and I share the following from his work:

- On average, men who smoke cut their lives short by 13.2 years.
- Women who smoke cut their lives short by 14.5 years.
- The number of teens smoking today has increased (The number of girls has especially increased; they might be smoking as a way to control weight.)
- There are serious smokers, and those who are social smokers are called "chippers"—people who smoke but are not yet addicted to nicotine. As they say, they can smoke 'em or leave 'em.

In the book, Gladwell describes the addicted serious smoker as someone who gets out of bed and lights up before his feet hit the ground. The British psychologist Hans Eysenck has argued that these serious smokers can be separated from non-smokers along very simple personality lines. He says the hard core smoker likes to be sociable, likes parties, has many friends, needs to have people to talk to, craves excitement, takes chances, and acts on the spur of the moment. Smokers prefer to keep moving and doing things, and they tend to be aggressive and lose their tempers quickly. The average smoking household spends seventy-three percent more on coffee and two to three times as much on beer as the average non-smoking household.

Interestingly, smokers also seem to be more honest about themselves than non-smokers. Smokers are relatively indifferent to what people think of them. These statistics Gladwell speaks of do not, of course, apply to all smokers. I do remember all the *fun* I had smoking, and indeed, I was perhaps more fun to be with when I smoked. (Ask some of my smoking girlfriends—)

Going Up in Smoke...

I thought I was perfectly happy and healthy smoking a pack a day for years. I actually smoked more than I wanted to admit. Let's face it—I loved to smoke. Mark Twain once said, "To cease smoking is the easiest thing I ever did. I ought to know; I've done it a thousand times." I knew I was killing myself but my smoking gave me smoke screens. I could hide my inner feelings and be with my friend—Cigẽ. I was living in the "N world"—a world of caffeINe, nicotINe, and wINe.

When I Tried to Quit, the "I's" Had It!

In my history of trying to quit, the "I's" had it. I scratched the patch and had horrible dreams. I had a small silver ball like a pierced earring placed in my earlobe, and each time I rubbed the small ball, it was to remind me not to smoke—it reminded me as I lit up.

I went to hypnosis with my friend Barb. We, of course, threw out our cigarettes during the session with great resolve and had to stop and pick up cigs for the two-hour drive home. I remember we did get a blue card saying if the hypnosis didn't seem to "take" the first time, we could use the coupon to try again. I threw it away when I opened my new pack of 100s.

Now I was excited. I had heard all the wonderful things about acupuncture. It was going to take care of so many obstacles for me. I went and had my session which was very relaxing, I thought, as I left the parking lot lighting up.

Finally, something worked. The Zyban was working. I had not smoked in nine months. I was so excited and proud about it that I did not renew my medication. I *knew* I was cured. I took my last pill on Friday morning, and by Sunday was buying my pack of cigarettes after church. You see, I had kept waiting to feel this new tremendous vim and vigor, which never came. I found myself sluggish, slow, and apathetic. When I lit up again, I was on a roll with more energy and enthusiasm to get things done. Amen! I was on a roll.

A few months later I ran into a friend whom I had not seen in almost a year. I knew she had quit smoking and chewed "the gum." I asked her how it was going. "Great," she said chewing like she was eating hay. Well, she was not smoking, but was now addicted to the nicotine gum. I thought I would at least give it a try. I did. I chewed the gum *and* smoked the cigarettes, knowingly inhaling 1500 poisons per cigarette.

I was reminded of a quote from Gertrude Stein, "Everybody gets so much information all day long that they lose their common sense." I realized the "I's" had it, and I continued to smoke cigarettes containing 250 toxic compounds including sixty carcinogens. And yet, the reality of the possible—and probable—impact of those carcinogens wasn't fazing me. Smoking for me was a performance. I was the "real me" when I was smoking. I was *fun!* Smoking was my friend, my companion, my all-purpose cleaner, fixer, and screener. Smoking was there for me in happiness, in sorrow, in anxiety, in fear, and in confidence. Smoking took care of all kinds of life situations.

Quitting is a Process, Not a Single Event

My only option left was to quit cold turkey. Everything else I had tried would not or had not worked for me. I am not saying that there aren't any programs and other cessation approaches that will work for folks; I just know what did *not* work for *me*. I had to face the cold hard reality and prepare for myself for the *process* of quitting.

The "I's" had it again. This time I knew it came in a form of a word I created: "WantItis." In the world of self-discipline, I knew I wanted to be smoke-free badly enough to be in the state of WantItis! The "I's" indeed had it. I needed to quit. I knew it was going to be hell for a while. I alerted friends and family: Beware—A woman without nicotine is a not a happy sight to behold or be with. I planned to divorce from the cigarette and to find a new light.

Writing Out My Plan

The most important question for me to answer was why I smoked. Why did I smoke? What were the symptoms, signs, and events that triggered my smoking? Why did I really want to quit? It was quite simple, yet very complicated. "Cigë" had been my friend for years, but I had decided the "divorce" was underway. The papers had been drafted and a quit date was set—a date that was printed on paper and in cement in my mind.

The next thing I did was make a list of the places and people I needed to avoid within the subsequent weeks if I was going to build up my own defenses. I needed to avoid the old haunts that housed the most vivid and enticing memories of smoking.

WantItis: Setting Yourself Up for Success, Not Failure

When I did commit to quit and began to practice WantItis, I was determined to set myself up for success, not failure. I did arrange my environment so I could execute new behaviors. I made a promise to myself that I would have passion about quitting, yet compassion for my very human self. I wrote down all the trigger spaces and places where I may, without thinking, want to light up. The list included all the triggers that beleaguered me from morning to night. I listed all of the times and places that prompted me to smoke during the day for years—in spite of my busy life. The list began with coffee, the phone, reading, writing, driving, and sitting. I fully realized how nicotine had been in control of me and of my life. That was a harsh reality that provoked a hollow echo of angry "I told you so's" within me. To battle them, I began to think clean air thoughts about how happy my musty lungs were going to feel smoke-free. I felt myself talking to them. They were now becoming a part of me I really wanted to take care of. I hoped in my heart of hearts that I was not too late

The "I's" Did It! I Quit!

I wrote *HOLY SMOKES* as I began the process of quitting. The statements that follow reflect my mood in the early days. They relate to my actions, my reactions, my anger for having to say goodbye to one of my best friends—a friend I had loved and enjoyed for many of the years of my life.

When I Did Quit, the "I's" Had It!

I practiced "yoga yawn." I took deep, deep breaths and yawned openly quite often in the light of day. I took forty-eight hours off from my life in general. I cleared my calendar for the Friday, Saturday, and Sunday that comprised the first three days of my official quitting process. I cloistered myself from everyone. My husband Bill was a godsend. I would and could not have done it without him. He was my coach and a believable coach because he is an ex-smoker himself. He was my cheerleader when I wanted to smoke. "Pat," he would say, "Just wait a few minutes. Move. Change your thinking. Change your life."

In many of my presentations now I have included that very simple phrase that helped me become smoke-free. (P.S. Here is a word to those of you who have a family or children and people who love you. Those people want what's best for you, too. They want you to quit. I am sure there are people who would help you out with the family in order to give you the best opportunity possible to fight this addiction in the first few terrible days.)

I think, in retrospect, that I created my own little miracle. It was so simple, yet so effective. I simply did the following:

A. Put a pack of cigarettes in the freezer so I'd know they were there—just in case.

B. Emptied all of the ashtrays and collected all of the butts.

C. Found a large, used coffee can, put the butts in, and added just the right amount of water.

D. Put the lid on the can and took it to the garage to simmer.

For the next week, every time I was home and thought I needed to smoke, I went out to the garage and lifted the lid. Need I say more about the odor? Needless to say, after one good whiff, the last thing I wanted was to smoke a cigarette!

I could not focus or concentrate in the first few days. I was suffering from a unique combination of FDD and ADD combined. I wanted to sleep. I knew that only time and positive thinking could take away my feeling of loss. I had put my cigarettes in the freezer and would go and just hold them. I know that sounds sick as I write about the experience now, but remember, I had just lost my best friend.

Of course, I wanted to eat and did to fill the hurt and the emptiness, that desperate feeling of loss. I developed an addiction to a whitening gum that was adding up to about $20 a day! I was in my favorite boutique called Jeanne's and my friend Gidget told me how my gum chewing was starting to annoy her. Well, she did not have to actually say it. Her body language told me first. It is nice to shop there because my friend Beckly helps me find clothes that do help hide the extra pounds which I am now losing.

I was attending my niece Kara's graduation from the University of South Dakota, having a nice time visiting and did notice the folks who had left the main reception area and went out on the deck to smoke. (You know, people who smoke at different meetings, conferences, and family gatherings adopt each other in a great ways and always feel closer in many ways. Well, I remained seated—proudly.) My brother Vincent sat down and started to talk about smoking and way to quit. He then handed me a white piece of plastic that was once a Comfort Inn pen. It was the same size as my 100's. He said, "Use it. It will work." Well, you know what? It did. I still carry that small piece of plastic as a reminder. It served me well—it was almost like an adult pacifier. At least, that's what it was for me.

The next week my brother Victor sent me his financial statement since going smoke-free in 1992. The statement indicated the money he had saved—an amount close to $24,000! I told people I had quit smoking and called ex-smokers for my nicotine fix just as folks look to each other for support in A.A. I quit drinking coffee the morning I quit smoking. I told myself a cigarette did not go well with oatmeal and milk. I also quit drinking any kind of alcohol. I knew myself too well. If I did have a few glasses of wine, I might just say to a friend, "Oh, give me one of those," and I would smoke it. We all know you only need to smoke one to be back on the smoking scene.

I began to drink a lot of water. Water, water, and more water. And a delightful drink called Irish green tea, a drink that my Grandmother Delia even approved. (Grandma never smoked and lived to be 100 years old. I am the second oldest in a family of ten children. My father smoked, but my mother never did. For years she was on the receiving end of secondhand smoke, but today she is eighty-seven years old and cancer-free! I think it's the prayers she has said.)

I ate pineapple every morning but would still wake up angry with myself for having smoked. You see, I would smoke in my dreams and, waking, I would be mad at myself for weakening. My husband Bill would tell me, "No, you did not smoke last night." That's part of the quitting process. You will dream about smoking for a few weeks. My real addiction now was not smoking but gum. I dropped the gum addiction, though, after my mouth had become so sore inside it was bleeding. To cool things down, I started eating Dream Bars. Oh, they are a wonderful sort of frozen treat (orange sherbet and vanilla ice milk) in a bar form. I would buy a carton of twelve bars and eat most of the carton in one night.

Now, that was a problem. Dream Bars were becoming my newest nightmare. I was just setting myself up for another addiction along the way. I finally addressed this new issue by simply not buying any more Dream Bars.

I started to live the "Four B's." I was headed for a breakdown, not a breakthrough. I had thought everything was going to be better when I quit smoking. Oh, I was wrong. I became bitter and brittle, ready to break into the B Land and ready to light up again. I needed to reflect on why I had quit smoking. I remembered a "Six-Pack" of instructions that I had written for my life years ago as part of an education course. My list of "A's" were: to be Attentive to my surroundings, to Accept who I was now in life, to be Aware of the blessings and the goodness around me, and to Appreciate and Affirm the best in myself, and to wrap myself in Accountability. I needed to reapply these thoughts daily to remind myself that God doesn't make junk and to continue to find that new light. I truly understood, "If it's going to be, it's up to me. I am. I can. I will, with the help of God."

Also, I understood that I couldn't fill the loss and the void with what I now call the Sad Five:

- Too much FOOD
- Too much SODA
- Too much BREAD
- Too much GUM
- Too much ICE CREAM

On the other hand, I needed to do the following:

- DO every day say out loud, "This is my choice. I am not going to smoke today. I do not know about tomorrow. Today I am not smoking. Take today. Take one step on the block and cut the worry. You are not at the corner." This cut the feeling of anxiety.
- DO take a deep breath. Yawn. Walk. Walk. Walk. Dance. Clean. (Cleaning provides visual and physical therapy.) Move your body. Write a prayer. Say it daily. Get an exercise ball. (These cost only about $20—less than a carton of cigarettes). Do treat yourself to things like new lotion, fresh flowers, a new candle, a new book about success and purpose.
- DO know that the risk of heart attack is lower, that your breath is cleaner. Know that your risk of cancer

is lower and that your hair smells fresher. Know that the risk of emphysema is lower, that your skin looks better, and that your health insurance is lower. Know that you no longer will waste time smoking. You will no longer look for exit signs in hotels and cafes. You will no longer look for potted plants to smoke behind!

When I quit smoking, eating less meat and eating more fruits and vegetables helped me, especially pineapple. I can't tell you why. It is truly mind over matter. We need to keep ourselves psyched about the dangers of smoking. I continued to check the water supply in my miracle bucket of cigarette butts and water in my coffee can in the garage. I cannot say enough about the positive effect that horrid odor had on my early success in becoming smoke-free. Just think of the investment—butts you have already smoked, a used container, and a little water. I do believe this was one of the most successful pieces to my homemade *"HOLY SMOKES* Cessation Program" by Pat. Daily—that can helped me to choose not to smoke—and days turned into weeks, weeks to months, and so on.

We are all imperfect human beings. If you do slip and smoke, don't beat yourself up mentally. Just begin anew. Do recognize that it takes time to change our behavior patterns. Know that quitting is a process—not a one-time event. Time helps us succeed. Write out a plan: Think it! Ink it! Live it! It truly works to write the plan down. You then own it. Change your thinking. Change your life. It's up to you!

My LIGHT Today: Living in Grateful Hope Today

Life is not what has been; it's what is in front of us. Whether we are sixteen or sixty, our lives are in front of us. What we choose to do determines our destiny. I no longer center myself on where I can smoke a quick cigarette. Instead, I am now living more in the moment, in the now. People are now my center—not smoking. I think of the wasted hours of smoking. Smoking is just a total waste of time, talent, and energy. I know I have become a better listener since becoming smoke-free.

Honor your body. God doesn't make junk! Your attitude toward your body literally impacts the atoms and molecules that comprise your body. "Happy thoughts make happy molecules." We have 20,000 connected moments a day in our minds. We need to make them positive. We need to be at peace with our bodies because our minds feed our souls. We cannot suffer from Giveupitis. We need to work for WantItis: I am, I can, I will. We need to daily choose not to give into, not to give up being smoke-free. I keep a journal—not a flower-covered book in which I write neatly—it's a yellow legal pad on I which free-write for positive mental health. "Did you know that 1,200 people die a day from smoke-related deaths? Smoke doesn't stay in the smoking section." These are just a couple of my entries.

Some Thoughts on a Morning Walk...

One morning as I was walking on the path of our athletic club, I was thinking about the fun I was missing out on now that I was no longer a "smoker." Remember, I had also quit drinking. I knew me, and if I was out socially and had a few glasses of wine, I was afraid I would let my guard down and smoke "just one." The strongest drink I now have is a great cup of dark java in the mornings. Funny, as I look back now, life is so much better when one no longer lives it in the "N World"—the world of nicotINe and wINe. I had to quit them both because in my life they went together. They went steady—they were "a couple."

In My Lifetime...

In my lifetime there have been some nice things happen to me and for me. I have taken much pride in my call, my purpose, and my mission in life. I don't think I have ever been so proud of me as I have been since becoming smoke-free. I share my smoking cessation prayer with you:

> Dear Lord, I can't do everything, yet I can do something. What I can do I will do. With your help, Lord, I will choose not to smoke today. Amen.

Some Things I Think About . . .

This is our last life as we know it. Age only matters if we are cheese. We need to paint or get off the ladder. My father Eddie would say it in a different way: Yes, you got it. Love yourself and forgive yourself because that makes room for you. Lead yourself to be the best version of you that you can be! Believe in yourself, and the magic will happen. Be kind and stay smoke-free. I share with you two of my favorite enrichments: "Start With Yourself" and "Different Drums and Different Drummers." I do not know the source of these two wonderful notes of instruction. However, I am grateful for their presence and influence in my life.

START WITH YOURSELF

The following words were written on the tomb of an Anglican Bishop (1100 A.D.) in the Crypts of Westminster Abbey: When I was young and free and my imagination had no limits, I dreamed of changing the world. As I grew older and wiser, I discovered the world would not change, so I shortened my sights somewhat and decided to change only my country. But it, too, seemed immovable. As I grew into my twilight years, in one last desperate attempt, I settled for changing only my family, those closest to me, but alas, they would have none of it. And now as I lie on my deathbed, I suddenly realize: If I had only changed myself first, then by example I would have changed my family. From their inspiration and encouragement, I would then have been able to better my country and, who knows, I may have even hanged the world.

Anonymous

DIFFERENT DRUMS
AND DIFFERENT DRUMMERS

If I do not want what you want, please try not to tell me that my want is wrong. Or if I believe other than you, at least pause before you correct my view. Or if my emotion is less than yours, or more, given the same circumstances, try not to ask me to feel more strongly or weakly. O yet if I act, or fail to act, in the manner of your design for action, let me be. I do not, for the moment at least, ask you to understand me. That will come only when you are willing to give up changing me into a copy of you. I may be your spouse, your parent, your offspring, your friend, or your colleague. If you will allow me any of my own wants, or emotions, or beliefs, or actions, then you open yourself, so that some day these ways of mine might not seem so wrong, and might finally appear to you as right – for me. To put up with me is the first step to under-

standing me. Not that you embrace my ways as right for you, but that you are no longer irritated or disappointed with me for my seeming waywardness. And in understanding me you might come to prize my differences from you and, far from seeking to change me, preserve and even nurture those differences.

HOLY SMOKES has come to an end. Yet, life is just really beginning again, for life's journey is the destination!

This is my cheer. I give the words to you—I have the actions. If I ever see you in person, I will teach you. I usually end most of my presentations with this very simple but important cheer:

> If it's going to be, It's up to me.
> I am.
> I can.
> I will.

LOUDER! LET'S HEAR YOU!

Blessings until we meet again.

About The Author

Pat McGill MA.Ed.

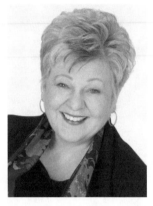

Pat McGill is founder and president of McGill Speaking and Training Resources. Pat works with organizations that want to create a more productive workplace where every employee is valued. Pat is a high content speaker and trainer who presents programs in a motivational style and tone. Pat's programs have been creating productive work places for businesses all over the country. Her high content, fun programs bring value to an organization's most precious resource—its employees. Pat brings a wide range of experiences in education, business, and administration. Pat has chaired many leadership positions in community, church, and educational associations.

Pat's most requested programs include: "Who Am I? Who Are You? Who Are We Together?" Women leaders: "Are You Worth Your Salt" "When Different is Good" Be Seated for Women" and "HOLY SMOKES"—a smoking cessation program. Clients have stated, "Pat brings an infectious 'can-do spirit' to all her presentations..."

Ms. McGill holds a Master's Degree of Education from St. Mary's University of Minnesota, she is a certified consultant for Inscape Publishing, an Adjunct Professor of Human Relations, a professional speaker, trainer, author, and columnist. Pat is a member of the National Speakers Association.

Pat McGill
McGill Speaking and Training Resources
352 Emerald Drive
Arnolds Park, Iowa 51331
Phone: 712.332.2965
Fax: 712-332-2965
Toll Free: 877.728.2557
Email: patmcgill@mchsi.com
www.patmcgill.net

Chapter 15

*"If all the tests are normal,
why don't I feel well?"*

Dr. Sherri J. Tenpenny

Kathi was worried. She had not felt well for months and had traveled from doctor to doctor, then specialist to specialist, seeking an explanation.

Instead of providing a definitive answer, each doctor had suggested a different diagnosis, many of which she could barely pronounce. In exchange for tens of thousands of dollars in tests and dozens of hours of time spread over many months, Kathi had received prescriptions for fifteen different drugs, but no answers.

Hoping to regain her health and wanting to be a "compliant" patient, she had dutifully purchased and taken all the medications. But instead of feeling better, each additional drug made her feel progressively worse.

With each passing month, she became more frustrated—and frightened. Not knowing why she felt so poorly was causing her imagination to run wild. The doctors had assured her she didn't have cancer, but could they be wrong? She had heard disturbing stories of people who weren't diagnosed until the cancer was far advanced. Could that be happening to her? The anxiety of not knowing what was wrong was nearly as taxing as her physical symptoms.

In fact, the entire conventional medical process had become disheartening. After months of following every suggestion her well-intended family doctor had made, Kathi concluded that conventional methods would not provide the solutions she needed.

Out of desperation she began searching the Internet for answers. There, she found support for the suspicions she had harbored all along – the medications she had been given were merely masking her symptoms, but quelling the symptoms was not the same as addressing the underlying *cause* of her problems.

After much deliberation, she decided to venture outside the "usual and customary" healthcare system and find an "alternative medicine doctor" to help her. But where would she find such a physician? And could that kind of doctor possibly do anything for her that had not already been tried by conventional medicine?

Stepping outside the box

Believing that word of mouth was the best way to proceed, Kathi asked friends if they could recommend a doctor who was familiar with alternative medicine. She was surprised at the responses, which ranged from, "You aren't serious?" to, "Do you think a 'voodoo doctor' can help you when The University Medical Center couldn't?" to "You know *those* aren't '*real doctors*' don't you?"

The disparaging reactions made her feel uneasy with her decision. Hoping to figure it out on her own, she decided to start her search at a health food store. Surely she could pick out a vitamin or two on her own, and find something more natural, so she could stop taking all those drugs.

As she drove across town, it occurred to her that she had never been in a health food store and wondered what she would encounter. Her friends had joked about the "Fruits and Nuts going to stores buy the fruits and nuts." She smiled as she thought of herself being placed in that category. As she turned into the parking lot, it occurred to her that the store was located in a rather affluent part of the city. Parking spaces were at a premium, but she eventually found a spot far from the door.

Walking past the rows of high-priced cars prior to entering the building, she noted that the atmosphere was upbeat and that the customers seemed genuinely happy to be there. "These people must know something I don't know...and they certainly don't look nutty to me," she mused.

As she strolled through the aisles, her eyes widened as she read the signs indentifying a medley of fruits, vegetables, and grains she had never heard of. She read the signs over the greens: "Basella rubra," "Bayam," "Bladder campion," and "beetberry." As she moved on, she saw bins of grains labeled "amaranth," "quinoa," and "buckwheat." Her curiosity was growing by the minute. "How do you cook these things? What do they taste like?" It slowly occurred to her that this was an entirely different world...and something she needed to learn more about.

Kathi spent most of the afternoon slowly winding her way through the aisles, mesmerized by the large number of food choices labeled "preservative free," "organically grown" and "farm raised." This was certainly a better way to eat! She rounded a corner and came to the section that housed the vitamins. "This is what I'm looking for," she thought confidently.

As her eyes scanned the shelves, her excitement quickly turned to dismay. She heard herself mutter, "I have no idea what these things are...how do I choose what's right for me?" The array of supplements on the shelves overwhelmed her even more than the large variety of bizarre vegetables she had passed earlier. She paid for the few items she had selected and left the store, resolving to find someone – a physician – to help her. But starting from scratch seemed simply overwhelming.

Back to the drawing board

As she drove home, Kathi become more determined than ever to find a doctor who "specialized" in alternative medicine. While at the health food store, she had met Sheila, a nice young woman who was working in the vitamin department. Sheila had offered her assistance, but Kathi had been too overwhelmed to know what questions to ask and too embarrassed to admit it. Perhaps Sheila could suggest a doctor? There was only one way to find out.

The following week, Kathi returned to the store feeling more assured than on her first visit. She headed directly to the vitamin section, hoping Sheila was on duty that day. She was in luck. As Kathi approached, the young woman smiled as she recognized the visitor.

"How can I help you today?" she asked pleasantly.

Kathi relaxed, introduced herself, and began to share her story of not feeling well, leading to many doctors and many pills, but no results. Sheila listened patiently while Kathi shared her long and frustrating tale.

"I've heard this story so many times before," Shelia replied empathetically. The kindness in her eyes and the softness of her voice reassured Kathi that Shelia was telling the truth. It was strangely comforting to know she was not the only person who had experienced these problems and frustrations.

"You really do need to see a doctor who can diagnose your problems before you begin randomly trying vitamins and supplements, Kathi," Sheila began. "Contrary to what your friends have told you, most doctors who include "alternative treatments" in their practices are fully licensed physicians who have undertaken extra courses beyond their medical school training. They call themselves 'Integrative Medicine specialists,' because they *integrate* both conventional medical tests and treatments with therapies you would consider to be 'alternative.'"

Kathi felt a twinge of hope.

"The phrase 'alternative medicine' has fallen into some disfavor because it implies an 'either/or' directive," Sheila continued. "Either you follow the instructions of your doctor and take the drugs that have been recommended *or* you throw all conventional medicine out the window and *just* take vitamins and herbs. Integrative medical doctors know you have to use *all* the available tools, even drugs at times, to tailor the treatment to the specific needs of the patient."

As Shelia spoke, the words resonated deep within Kathi. She knew she was in the right place, and she was suddenly overcome with emotion. Tears welled up as she asked, "Where can I find an Integrative Medicine doctor? Is there someone you would recommend?"

With confidence, Sheila replied, "I have heard nothing but good things about the doctors at the Integrative Medicine Clinic across town called OsteoMed II. I think you would be very pleased with your care there."

"That is right near my house!" Kathi exclaimed.

"Even better," Sheila replied softly.

Finding a doctor at last

Kathi rushed home to tell her husband the news. She was very hopeful that she was finally on the right path. Perhaps in addition to an accurate diagnosis, she could even get well – and without medications. That afternoon, Kathi located the phone number for OsteoMed II in the yellow pages. Excitedly, she called for an appointment. A pleasant voice answered the phone. "Hello, my name is Natalie. How can I help you?"

Kathi explained that she would like to make a new patient appointment as soon as possible with the doctor. Natalie's response startled and disheartened Kathi. The first available appointment was six weeks away.

Natalie politely asked, "Are you familiar with the services we offer?"

"Not really," Kathi replied. "But I was referred to your Clinic by Sheila from the health food store, and she thought the doctor there could help me."

The receptionist chuckled softly and said, "We have three doctors, and yes, Sheila refers a lot of patients to us because she has seen the results. Let me tell you a bit about our Clinic."

For the next ten minutes, Kathi learned about the types of diagnostic tests and treatments available at the Clinic. Although the unique processes that involved blood, saliva, hair, urine, and stool testing sounded very interesting, many things Natalie described were completely foreign to Kathi: Kinesiology? Muscle testing? Homeopathy? Detoxification? Again, she realized she had a lot to learn.

"Do you accept my form of insurance"? Kathi inquired.

"Unfortunately, we do not participate with any insurance companies," Natalie explained. "Our doctors believe that part of getting well involves taking ownership in the healing process, and paying directly for your care is part of that process. We give you a receipt, called an 'HCFA form,' to send to your insurance company. Most of our patients get from twenty-five to eighty percent of their costs reimbursed from their health insurance companies. We do what we can to help you with that."

Wow, this really is different, Kathi thought to herself. "I'll have to talk this over with my husband. But in the meantime, can I make an appointment? I want to get on your schedule since it seems your doctors are very busy."

"Certainly. We will send you a patient packet that has more information about the Clinic and forms that we ask you to complete prior to your appointment. We suggest that you set aside at least one and a half hours to fill them out as completely as possible. I highly suggest you take a look at our website before you see the doctor. There is a lot more information there about us. Is there anything else that I can answer for you today?"

That evening, Kathi relayed to her husband how polite Natalie had been while confidently answering her questions about the Clinic. She was impressed with how unrushed the conversation had been—quite different from calling her family doctor's office for a routine appointment!

Together, Kathi and Tom intensely reviewed the information on the Clinic's website for more than an hour. Eventually, she broached the topic of fees, feeling a bit nervous about telling Tom that treatments at the Clinic may not be covered by their health insurance.

"Kathi, our insurance company has paid many thousands of dollars for you to have dozens of tests and see many doctors who haven't helped you one bit," he responded. "If we need to take funds from our savings for you to get well, and if these new doctors can help you, how much is that worth? Are you going to make an appointment?"

Kathi jumped up and threw her arms around Tom's neck in excitement. "I have an appointment in six weeks!" she exclaimed. She knew she was on her way to getting well.

Common ground

If this story resonates with you, you're not alone. Tens of thousands of Americans are searching for help beyond the scope of conventional medicine. Dr. David Eisenberg's landmark study was the first to document that expenditures for alternative medicine professional services were conservatively estimated to be $21.2 billion in 1997, with at least $12.2 billion paid out-of-pocket.[1] It is assumed that the numbers have increased substantially since that time.

The most comprehensive and reliable findings to date on Americans' use of alternative medicine are from the National Center for Complementary and Alternative Medicine (NCCAM) and the National Center for Health Statistics (NCHS, part of the Centers for Disease Control and Prevention). According to a nationwide government survey released in May, 2004, 74.6 percent of U.S. adults age eighteen years and older (31,044 surveyed) had

---

1 Eisenberg, D. M., et. al. *Trends in alternative medicine use in the United States, 1990-1997: results of a follow-up national survey. JAMA.* November 11, 1998;280(18):1569-75.

used some form of alternative healing in their life, and just over sixty-two percent had used Complementary/Alternative Medicine (CAM) in the preceding year.[2]

The survey revealed that people tried alternative methods for a wide array of diseases and conditions. The most common included: painful conditions in the back, neck, head, or joints; colds and flu; anxiety or depression; gastrointestinal disorders; or sleeping problems.

Although most people surveyed chose to use alternative medicine along with conventional medicine rather than in place of it, the following reasons were stated for using CAM (more than one could be selected):

- Health would improve more when used in combination with conventional medical treatments (55%)
- CAM would be interesting to try (50%)
- Conventional treatments did not help (28%)
- Conventional medical treatments were too expensive (13%)

Of particular interest, 26% of the respondents indicated that a conventional medical professional had suggested that the patient try CAM.[3] Many patients have reported that their physician, whom they had ordinarily found to be caring, thoughtful, and understanding became angry, defensive, and dismissive when the possibility of using alternative therapies was even mentioned.[4] This caused nearly 70% of patients to not tell their conventional practitioner about this use.[5] This distinct change in attitude and acceptance of alternative methods by conventionally trained physicians will benefit both practitioners and patients.

Perhaps the most important reason physicians are changing their perceptions about non-mainstream medical therapies is that an extensive amount of research is now published each month in

---

[2] *The Use of Complementary and Alternative Medicine in the United States.* Barnes, P., Powell-Griner, E., McFann, K., Nahin, R. *CDC Advance Data Report #343. Complementary and Alternative Medicine Use Among Adults: United States,* 2002. Released May 27, 2004: http://nccam.nih.gov/news/camsurvey_fs1.htm.

[3] Ibid.

[4] Gordon, J., 1996. "Alternative medicine and the family physician." *American family physician,* 54(7):2205-12.

[5] Jonas, W., 1998. "Alternative medicine and the conventional practitioner." *JAMA,* 279(9):708-9.

mainstream medical journals on the use of nutritional supplements for health and healing. One of the best publications available to demonstrate this is *The Clinical Pearls*. This monthly newsletter extracts 15 to 30 research articles each week from peer-reviewed, mainstream, conventional medical journals and prints summaries for review. The company offers a free service to search its extensive database containing more than 10,000 articles compiled from 1989 to the present, at www.Vitasearch.com. Doctors can no longer claim "there is no proof" or "there is no research on alternative medicine" because voluminous amounts of studies have been completed, and published, on the benefits of nutrients.[6]

Incorporating nutrition into a medical practice is usually the first step in becoming an Integrative Medicine physician. However, moving beyond that point, and learning to view the entire body as a "whole" can be difficult. Medical school training leads to the development of specialties and subspecialties in which physicians become experts on an increasingly limited portion of the body. Ironically, in an age of specialization, greater responsibility is being placed on the patient to determine the underlying cause of his own health problems.

Key concepts in Integrative Medicine for everyone

Everyone needs a basic understanding of how his or her body is put together and how it functions. After all, we each have only *one body* to last an entire lifetime. How many cars, houses, and jobs do we have in comparison? Having a better understanding of the major components of the body, and how they work, will help you participate in the process of restoring and maintaining your health.

Unlike conventional medicine, the discipline referred to as "Integrative Medicine" has a core set of principles used to identify and treat the underlying causes of a wide variety of health problems. To illustrate the use of these principles, I have developed a simple model to explain the core components of the body and how they are interrelated. Once you see how the components work, you will understand why an Integrative Medicine model for

---

[6] For more information on *Clinical Pearls News,* go to
http://www.prescription2000.com

health and healing is markedly different from the way conventional medicine is practiced.

The following diagram represents the "house" you live in, called "Your Body." Like your body, the house diagram is composed of the core components, I call "boxes." Refer to this diagram frequently throughout this discussion to easily understand how the "House Model for Integrative Medicine" is applied to health and healing.

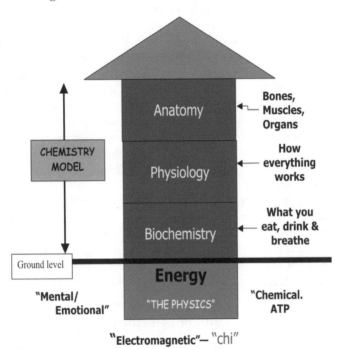

"Your Body's House", ©2001
New Medical Awareness Seminars, LLC
www.NMAseminars.com

This model represents the "house" you live in called your Body. Every human's "house" is constructed with the same components, the same "set of boxes." The boxes contain "anatomy," "physiology," and "biochemistry," the major structural subsets of each human. The box representing the foundation, or basement, is labeled "energy."

Similar to the physical house you live in, the "basement" of your human house is out of sight, taken for granted, yet structurally, it's the most important component of a sound building. We'll soon see why having a healthy "energy component" is critically important for overall health.

A closer look at the "floors" of the house

The top floor, or box, of the house is anatomy, referring to the structural components of the body. Anatomy is the body's "framework" – the skin, organs, muscles, and bones. The anatomy "box" is purposefully placed on the "top floor" because it is the most visible, and forms our individual look and identity.

Anatomy is directly supported by physiology, the second box. Simply put, physiology is "how everything in the body works" – processes such as digestion and absorption of nutrients, the mechanics of respiration, and the removal of wastes. Physiological processes differentiate living from non-living organisms. Without physiology, anatomy is not a living creation. Even a rock has anatomy (framework) but it certainly doesn't have physiology (living processes).

The next supporting "box" is biochemistry, an intimidating word, until explained in its simplest terms. Biochemistry is what we eat, drink, and breathe, including the vitamins and supplements we take and the drugs we consume. Nutrients are on the "ground floor" of the house because food, water, and nutrition are the vital components needed by the physiology to drive the anatomy.

The body's physics: real and not-so-subtle

Just like the brick-and-mortar house you live in, your body's "house" rests on a foundation. The body's "foundation box" labeled "energy" is shown at the base of the model by design, because energy supports the entire body/house. A well-functioning energy compartment is the most important part of health. This is the area of the body that is commonly overlooked by Western medicine when attempting to diagnose and treat disease.

Many people are uncomfortable with the concept of the body's "energy" or the term "energy medicine." I have observed patients who were initially wary of energy medicine, referring to it as "Eastern" or "mystical" and even calling it "un-Christian."

Accessing the body's "energetic forms" for diagnosis and healing is not a matter of theology. It is not about a "belief," as in, "I don't believe in energy medicine." Energy medicine is treating the "other half of the body," which is composed of chemistry *and* physics. With a more thorough explanation, most patients understand that energy medicine evaluates a segment of the body—the body's physics – overlooked by all of conventional medicine. It is about health and healing at the most basic level and is neither "mysterious" nor "mystical."

Evaluating the body's energy patterns requires a different diagnostic tool than we are familiar with using. We are comfortable assessing the body's chemistry through blood, urine, hair, and saliva specimens. We should find equal comfort with the tests and equipment used to access and treat the body's bio-electrics, or physics.

A short history of energy devices

In the early 1950s, Reinhold Voll, a German medical doctor, developed a testing device to electrically locate acupuncture points. He successfully demonstrated that these points, known to Chinese acupuncturists for millennia, had a different resistance measurement to a tiny electrical current passed through the body than did the adjacent tissues. These machines, known as "Electroacupuncture According to Voll" (EAV) devices, introduce a low voltage electrical charge into the body and then measure the precise amount of electric current conducted through known acupuncture points. The electromagnetic imprints of various substances can also be introduced, or tested, with the EAV device and useful diagnostic information can be elicited by the trained user.

A full explanation of this technology is beyond the scope of this discussion[7], but it should be known that EAV technologies, also referred to "Meridian Stress Assessment (MSA) instruments," have been utilized widely for more than 35 years throughout Europe and in other parts of the world. MSA instruments have been manufactured in Germany, Japan, China, France, Denmark,

---

[7] For a well written discussion on The History of Meridian Stress Assessment, go to http://www.biomeridian.com/web/meridian-stress-assessment.htm

Russia, and more recently in the United States. The technology, however, has only been available for a few years in this country.

The body's energy: more than one

The body is composed of a variety of different energy types. Our model contains three basic energy categories: chemical, mental/emotional, and electromagnetic. Chemical energy in the body is stored in a molecule called adenosine triphosphate (ATP). All of the food we eat is metabolized through complex physiological processes resulting in the creation of ATP—the body's "gasoline." This molecule is essential for life; when the production of ATP stops, we literally die.

Mental/emotional energy connects our feelings with our body. We readily perceive this type of energy when we are happy and excited – the body feels a sense of well being and delight. Our heart rate accelerates, we can't sit still, and our mind races with a variety of unrelated thoughts. Conversely, when sad or grieving, our body can lose its appetite, experience insomnia, and even manifest a variety of unrelated physical symptoms.

Recognizing this, we accept that our emotions, a form of energy, have a powerful effect on our anatomy and physiology. We have heard many stories of persons who were healed from illness ranging from psychosis to cancer by resolving long-standing emotional conflicts. An energy shift occurred in the "foundation" that manifested through the rest of the "house," repairing "structural flaws within the "upper floors" that had been the focus of previous suppressive treatments using drugs.

Suppose that your physical house has a second story window that leaked (i.e. the problem appears to be in the "physiology box"). Every year, you replace the window but it continues to leak. You grow increasingly frustrated because you have had countless carpenters (doctors) evaluate the problem (repeated blood tests and x-rays) and many have made recommendations that should have corrected the problem.

However, with each new recommendation (each new drug), the windows not only continued to leak but leaked worse than before! Eventually, you hire a construction engineer (integrative medicine doctor) to take a look at the *entire* house. He or she discovers that the problem has nothing to do with the windows! The real problem was a structural flaw in your "basement" that involved the "foundation" of your house (disruptions in the physics part of your body). You had been looking in the wrong "box" for the solution (diagnosis and treatment). Once the "cause" was clearly identified, the "cure" was long lasting.

The most important energy: *Chi*

Even more powerful than the chemical energy (ATP) and the mental/emotional energy, which comprise a part of the physics "foundation", is the third type of energy, the "life force energy" existing in the body's electromagnetic core. Practitioners of ayurvedic medicine call this energy 'prahna.' In Chinese medicine, it is referred to as *'chi.'* These subtle energies are powerful, measurable and all encompassing, meaning, "the whole is greater than the sum of the parts."

Electricity that travels through the wires of your physical house can't be seen or felt. It has no color, taste, or smell. We can experience its presence, however, by turning on a "light switch." The energy that traverses your body's house courses along channels called meridians and can be activated by stimulating the channel's corresponding acupuncture point. Acupuncture points and the acupuncture meridians have been identified and mapped by Electro Dermal Screening (EDS) equipment. What is interesting is that abnormal EDS measurements identified at a known acupuncture point correlate with abnormalities found within the point's corresponding organ.[8]

Unfortunately, most conventional physicians are not familiar with EAV devices, and because they are not universally accepted by conventional medicine, EAV testing is not covered by conventional medical insurance. This is a Catch 22: if EAV devices were reimbursed by insurance, there would be a rush for the doctors to learn about – and purchase – the machines for their practices. But until doctors accept its use, EAV will not be researched and will not be covered by insurance. The current system seems to ensure that unconventional/unfamiliar devices used in Energy Medicine will remain under utilized.

Is this energy medicine "weird" medicine?

I have had many opportunities to speak to groups of conventionally trained medical doctors and have explained the

---

[8] Tsuei J., Lam F., Chou P. "Clinical applications of the EDST." IEEE Eng Med Biol 1996;15:3:67-75.

importance of using the concepts described in the "house diagram model" to care for their patients. When I reached the section of the presentation that describes the "energy" in the body, I have often felt the "energy" in the room shift, from acceptance to resistance, until I point out that they have been "energy medicine doctors" throughout their professional lives. They just haven't framed it in those terms. After the scoffing subsides, I go on to defend my statement.

Physicians order tests every day that measure the energy of the body: an EKG measures the electricity, or energy, of the heart; an MRI (which stands for Magnetic Resonance Imaging) evaluates the electromagnetic charges emitted from tissues and then converts the energy into a picture through sophisticated software; an EEG, ordered to detect the presence of seizure activity, measures the electromagnetic impulses, the physics, of the brain; and so forth. These common technologies, along with many others, are used to measure the large, or macroscopic, energy patterns within the body. At that point, many of the physicians start to have an internal "shift," an opening to the possibility that there is more to this "energy stuff" than they had previously considered

A key difference

What sets most Integrative Medicine physicians apart is that they understand that by identifying and correcting the body's disrupted energy imbalances *first,* many of the symptoms within the "upper floors" of the body's house can improve or resolve spontaneously. Deficient biochemistry leads to dysfunctional physiology and poorly operating anatomy. Symptoms originate because something is missing biochemically, leading to faulty physiological and anatomical functioning.

A symptom is a "warning sign" that something is wrong and needs attention. Here's an analogy: you walk into your house at the end of the day to discover that your smoke alarm is shrieking. Instead of scrambling to look for the fire, you yank the battery from the detector and toss it in the trash, mumbling, "What an annoying sound that thing makes!"

When you develop hypertension, chronic diarrhea, or allergic symptoms, your body is giving you a "warning sign" that something is awry. Simply masking the symptom with a drug—without closely examining all the "boxes" for the cause—is no different

than disabling your smoke alarm without bothering to look for the fire.

A real life story

The validity and usefulness of this model became clear to me when I had a real life problem with my physical house.

I was planning to move to Cleveland and listed my house for sale with a local realtor, a friend of mine. I was excited to meet him after work the day he had shown the first couple through my house. My excitement quickly faded when I saw the look on his face. I knew better than to ask if they were interested in making an offer.

"Sherri, do you know that none of the doors in the second story of your house close?" he asked with concern. Obviously, I had no idea this was a problem. I lived alone and never had the occasion to close the upstairs doors. I hurried home and was distressed to find that not only did the doors not close, but that the mismatch was more than three-eighths of an inch! I knew I had a serious – and potentially expensive – problem that needed attention before anyone could (or should) purchase my house.

The following day, I spoke to a construction engineer. After explaining the situation in detail, she asked, "Do you also have large cracks in your walls?"

"As a matter of fact, I do," I cautiously replied, concerned this was suddenly becoming a larger and more costly problem than already anticipated. I was hoping for a referral to a carpenter, and now I also needed someone who could repair plaster!

Her next question surprised me. She asked, "What kind of problems do you have in your basement?"

"I don't know," I replied. "My house has a crawlspace. The house was built in a new neighborhood, and I have never gone down there." Concerned, she agreed to come to my house the next day and take a look.

Nervously, I waited for her to arrive. After a quick tour through the house, she had solved the puzzle. "There's your problem," she said, pointing to the upstairs loft. My eyes followed her finger up the stairs to the solid oak, ceiling-to-floor bookcases I had installed on the north and east sides of the loft shortly after I had moved in, and promptly loaded with more than a half-ton of books. The ground was still soft beneath the foundation and the house was tipping over, literally!

After "diagnosing" the underlying cause of the problem, she descended into the crawlspace and designed a plan to straighten the house. Her team installed a jack and once a week someone came to the house to turn the crank and insert a small wedge of wood. After about six weeks, the doors closed easily on their hinges and the wall cracks seem to seal themselves. Eventually, I sold the house and moved to Cleveland without a hitch.

The moral of the story?

The "house doctor" knew "which box to look in" and found the "real" problem in the foundation, not on the second story loft where the "obvious" problem was. I could have hired a carpenter and a plaster specialist, but that would only have addressed the "symptoms" it would not have fixed the problem. The solution was to fix the foundation.

Disruptions in the energy—the key to patient evaluation

The top three floors described in your body's house exist above "ground level" and are considered to be the "chemistry model" of Western medicine. When symptoms occur, the doctor looks for problems in the anatomy by using a variety of x-rays and in the physiology through many different blood tests. If an abnormality is found, a "correction" is attempted by prescribing a biochemical drug. This may alleviate the symptom but it certainly doesn't identify or correct the cause of the problem. This is where conventional medicine and Integrative Medicine have distinctly different ways of evaluating and treating ailments.

Certainly, Integrative Medicine physicians may recommend x-rays and blood tests when necessary. However, these physicians utilize a variety of other tests that evaluate the functional status of the body. For example, if the patient's symptoms suggest underlying adrenal stress, a conventional doctor would order a blood cortisol level. An Integrative Medicine doctor would order a saliva test that collects a series of four samples over the course of the day: upon rising, at noon, at dinner, and at bedtime. The value of this cannot be over-stated because cortisol measurements should be highest in the morning and lowest before retiring. An isolated sample—blood or saliva—during the day has no clinical value. This is one example of unique "functional medicine tests" used by Integrative Medicine physicians.

However, where Integrative Medicine physicians excel is in evaluating disruptions in the physics of the body, in the "energy box." As previously described, devices such as the EAV and Meridian Stress Assessment are available for testing the energy level at acupuncture points by measuring skin resistance.[9] Another tool is available for quickly evaluating the body's energy system without using a machine. This technique is called muscle testing, also known as kinesiology.

Kinesiology—a tool for the testing the physics

Developed in the early 1970s by Dr. George Goodheart and termed "Applied Kinesiology," muscle testing has evolved into a variety of forms and uses.

The fundamental principle behind muscle testing is that placing a substance on the body that it perceives to be harmful can weaken a muscle. Conversely, introducing a substance to the body's energy field that the body perceives to be beneficial, or of no harm, can strengthen a muscle. Most significantly, the test subject does not need to know what the test substance is for the muscle to be tested as "strong" or "weak." What is being tested involves our "subtle kinesthetic sense"—the body's subtle energy/physics.

Unlike our physical senses, our subtle kinesthetic sense is "non-organic." We have eyes to see, ears to hear, a nose to smell, a tongue to taste, and skin to feel, but no specific organ is responsible for our kinesthetic sense. It operates independently from our other senses and thoughts. Our kinesthetic "memory" records every food, plant, mineral, animal, person, and chemical we have encountered since the day we were born. A full appreciation of this ability of our body falls into the realm of quantum physics, far beyond the scope of this discussion. We know, however, there is much more to our universe and our body's senses than "what meets the eye." Muscle testing is a way to superficially tap into our body's "physics box," and identify disruptions that can cause a myriad of health conditions not detected in the "chemistry box."

---

[9] Radin, D. I. "A possible proximity effect on human grip strength. Percept Mot Skills." 1984 Jun;58(3):887-8.

Questions arise regarding the validity and reproducibility of muscle testing. One book that discusses this in detail is, "Afterwards, You're A Genius: Faith, Medicine, and the Metaphysics of Healing" by Chip Brown. Brown, an award winning writer who has written for the Washington Post, The New Yorker, and others, uses a combination of scientific fact and humor to explain how energy medicine works. Reviews of the book are available at www.amazon.com.

Brown mentions a study published in 1984 by D. I. Radin called, "A possible proximity effect on human grip strength." Brown states, "He [Radin] looked into applied kinesiology, a fringe diagnostic technique based on the theory that muscle strength reflects the body's sensitivity to various substances. Radin ran double blind and triple blind trials with fifty-eight adults using vials of sugar and sand and a dynometer that measured the gripping strength of the hand. The results startled him and he noted that they seemed 'preposterous.' But data was data, and his data showed that muscle strength decreased significantly when subjects held vials of sugar."[10]

The most common disruption identified by using muscle testing to examine the "energy box" is the presence of food allergies. The notion that food allergies can cause medical illness is the basis of much controversy. Most articles in conventional medical literature state that true food allergy is rarely a cause of a patient's symptoms. Because food allergies can produce many different symptoms in different organ systems simultaneously, most traditional physicians have difficulty understanding and accepting this concept.

The House Model easily explains away this resistance: It is because they are not looking in the correct "box." Food allergy disruptions are most readily identified in the "energy box" causing a myriad of symptoms in all the other "floors of the house." If you spend the day cleaning out drawers looking for your car keys, but they are really in your coat pocket, you won't find the keys because you are not looking in the right "box."

---

[10] Radin, D. I. "A possible proximity effect on human grip strength. Percept Mot Skills." 1984 Jun;58(3):887-8.

Allergy confusion—choosing a better word

Much of the misunderstanding that comes from suggesting food allergies can cause health problems is centered on the word *"allergy."* The word "allergy" is derived from two Greek words meaning, "altered reaction." When Western medicine began to scientifically research allergic response in the human body in the 1930s, a biochemical pathway was discovered that involved a protein found in our blood that was named IgE—immunoglobulin type E. This antibody is responsible for causing the symptoms we recognize as allergic reactions: sneezing, itching, watery nose, etc. It is this definition of "allergy," associated with an IgE-mediated response, that is accepted by the medical community. Typically, IgE-mediated food reactions occur within minutes to several hours after exposure to an allergen. If an immediate and readily identifiable reaction—such as diarrhea (a reaction to lactose), or anaphylaxis (a reaction to peanuts) occurs, then conventional medicine accepts this as a "food allergy."

A second type of immunoglobulin, known as IgG, can mediate food and environmental reactions (more often referred to as "sensitivities"). These reactions, called "delayed-type reactions," can occur up to seventy-two hours after an exposure. Unfortunately, this does not fit into the classic "allergy" format caused by IgE immunoglobulins. Subsequently, the concept of delayed food, environmental, and chemical allergies has been very difficult for the medical community to accept.

A pilot study published in 1998 attempted to determine whether subjective muscle testing can prospectively determine those individuals with specific hyperallergenic responses.

Seventeen subjects showed muscle-weakening (inhibition) reactions to oral provocative testing. This was considered a "positive response" by using Applied Kinesiology (A.K.) muscle testing as a screening procedure and indicated that the person had a food hypersensitivity (allergy) to the food. Serum tests were then performed using both a RAST test (radio-allergosorbent test) and immune complex test for IgE and IgG. Serum tests confirmed 19 of the 21 food allergies (90.5 percent) suspecte, based on the applied kinesiology screening procedures.

The study offers a basis to examine further a means by which to predict the clinical utility of using a neuromuscular response to a given substance for a given patient.

269

Acute vs. Delayed reactions: Hidden causes of problems

Because delayed food reactions are almost always "hidden" and difficult to identify, symptoms may not emerge until long after eating the causative foods. Hidden food sensitivities have become the cause of many common, chronic, and incapacitating illnesses.

To complicate the process even further, several foods may be causing different symptoms at the same time. Hence, a patient may complain of symptoms that include headaches, abdominal cramping, and wheezing, and appear to be suffering from a puzzling illness. The doctor generally attempts to identify separate causes for these complaints (i.e., ordering x-rays, blood tests and the prescribing a variety of drugs) when the common denominator is frequently complex food allergy causing all of these symptoms *simultaneously*.

The good news

Fortunately, an Integrative Medical physician, schooled in energy medicine and trained in muscle testing, will know to look in the "energy box" to identify hidden food allergies not diagnosed by conventional testing. Since the body "remembers" a previous sensitivity through its kinesthetic memory, muscle testing can identify the specific substance that is causing symptoms upon recurrent exposure. After the substance is identified, an energy treatment – tapping on specific acupuncture points along the spine and on the arms and legs – is used to change the kinesthetic memory. A new "memory" is imprinted and the next time the substance is introduced, the body no longer reacts to the substance. Delayed reactions stop, the symptoms resolve and the body heals. It is as simple as knowing how to look in the "energy box" and knowing how to use an "energy tool" to repair the cause of the problem.

The Day of the appointment arrives

The six weeks Kathi waited for her appointment to see the Integrative Medicine doctor seemed like an eternity. Deciding to make good use of the time, Kathi did her homework. She completed the medical history forms she had received in the mail in detail, and again reviewed the clinic's website and listened to the audiotape that came with her introductory packet on allergy elimination. Much focus was placed on a process referred to as "muscle testing," another new concept for Kathi, She researched the technique on the Internet and read the suggested book, *The Food Allergy Cure*, by Dr. Ellen Cutler.

It had never occurred to Kathi that many of her symptoms – irritable bowel, daily headaches, eczema, extreme fatigue and others – could all have a single, related cause: unrecognized and untreated food and environmental allergies! None of the doctors at the University Medical Center had even suggested this as a possible cause.

She arrived early for her appointment, with a mixed sense of excitement and apprehension. She was pleasantly surprised by the décor of the office. Not only was it much larger than she had expected, but also very modern, clean, and comfortable. The classical music and well-kept, colorful aquarium were welcoming touches. The receptionist greeted her warmly and within minutes she was taken to a well-appointed and pleasant examining room. After a short interview by the assistant, the doctor arrived and she was once again greeted with a reassuring, welcoming handshake.

"Good morning, Kathi," the doctor began. "We are glad you're here and we look forward to working with you. What can I help you with today?"

She thought she would be controlled, but all the months of seeking an answer and weeks of waiting for the appointment pushed her to her limit. Unexpectedly, Kathi burst out, "I have been going to the University Medical Center for months. I have had every possible test and taken dozens of pills that made me worse instead of better. If all the tests are normal, how can I possibly be this sick?"

Smiling knowingly, the doctor calmly replied, "Kathi, we have heard this so many times before. Why don't you tell me more about how you are feeling, and we'll see if we can't find something that hasn't been tried before."

From there, Kathi was given the opportunity to explain her detailed medical history and ask her full list of questions, without once feeling rushed or being interrupted. The doctor was fully attentive and obviously interested in what she described. This was certainly a different experience!

After nearly an hour, the doctor said, "Kathi, I am quite confident we can help you. We have treated many people from all over the country—29 states and 4 foreign countries actually-- with similar problems. I have developed my own method of allergy elimination called 'Sensitivity Reduction Technique, or SRT®.' We have used SRT® to eliminate problems with asthma, acid reflux, ADHD, and even hormonal difficulties. From your symptoms, I suspect that you have a number of underlying, unrecognized food and environmental allergies we refer to as 'sensitivities.' Are you familiar with muscle testing?"

"Well, sort of. I read the books you suggested and listened to your tape. I think I understand the concept, at least," Kathi eagerly replied.

"That's good! I will introduce you to my assistant. We will get you tested and go from there. You'll probably be surprised by what we find."

As it turned out, muscle testing revealed Kathi had sensitivities to eggs, dairy, fructose, white sugar, white flour, corn, wheat, and several other foods. Kathi *was* surprised... and relieved. Perhaps this *was* the answer after all!

The assistant proceeded with the SRT® treatment, which involved obtaining a small vial of blood from a finger-stick, and the simulation of specific acupuncture points in her back, arms, and legs with a small tapping instrument. She was asked to recline on a comfortable table for fifteen minutes.

During the rest period, Kathi noted warm sensations that seemed to wash over her body. The pleasant music relaxed her; she nearly fell asleep. A timer announced the end of the treatment. Then, as instructed, she went to the checkout area for further instructions.

As Kathi drove home, she became aware of an overall sense of well being that she hadn't experienced in years. The drive gave her the opportunity to reflect on what she had learned during the preceding two months. She affirmed the amount of determination it had taken to overcome the warnings of her friends and she felt a twinge of pride at her strength. "The process of 'getting well' is completely different than the conventional practice of 'managing my symptoms,'" she reasoned. She had a new insight regarding getting well: achieving it is a matter of personal responsibility. She resolved to go to the health food store early next week to thank Sheila with a huge hug for suggesting that she go to OsteoMed II .

She turned into her driveway, eager to share her exciting good news with Tom. She was sure the clinic was the right place and the right choice. She was on her way to recovery.

Recommended reading:

The Food Allergy Cure, by Ellen Cutler, D.C., M.D.
Winning the War Against Asthma & Allergies by Ellen Cutler, D.C.
Say Goodbye to Illness by Devi Nambudripad, D.C., L.Ac., R.N., Ph.D.

About The Author

Dr. Sherri J. Tenpenny

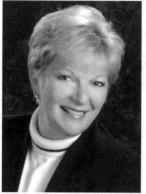

Dr. Sherri J. Tenpenny is the President and CEO of OsteoMed II, an Integrative Medicine clinic established in 1996 in Ohio to create a different type healthcare experience for patients. Trained as an osteopathic physician, she understands that the body has the ability to heal without drugs when the "missing components" are replaced. The physicians at OsteoMed II have been trained to use her model, "Your Body's House™" to treat both chemistry and physics in the body. Thousands have come to OsteoMed II from across the country to regain their health. Highly respected, entertaining and informative, Dr. Tenpenny is asked to speak at major conferences throughout the year in the US and abroad, and is a regular guest on radio talk shows and TV programs. She has published investigative reports for national magazines, newspapers and Internet news sites, including www.mercola.com, the #1 health news site on the web, and www.RedFlagsDaily.com, the highly respected health science site. Dr. Tenpenny is also an outspoken advocate for free choice regarding vaccination. In addition to topics on Integrative Medicine, she is invited to present her extensive research on vaccination hazards, warnings that are rarely portrayed by conventional medicine, at meetings around the world. Her two DVDs, "Vaccines: The Risks, Benefits and Choices" and "Vaccines: What CDC and Science Documents Reveal" have helped thousands of parents make an informed choice regarding vaccination. These two presentations contain a combined five hours of extensively researched facts gleaned from conventional medical journals. Married and passionately devoted to her business partner/mate, her personal life goal is to travel the world while sharing information on a "better way" to be and stay healthy.

OsteoMed II
7251 Engle Road, #250
Middleburg Heights, Ohio 44130
Phone: 440.239.3438
Fax: 440.238.3440

www.osteomed.com
www.nmaseminars.com
www.novaccines.com

Chapter 16

Imagine...

Donna Collins

Imagine that you could manifest whatever you want.
Imagine that you could focus during meditations or visualizations.
Imagine that you could tap into your best and highest destiny.

It all started with my new house. Nestled in the woods, resting by a creek, my new house had olive green coffeepot and frying pan wallpaper in the kitchen—not exactly what I had imagined. So I subscribed to all the interior design magazines available and when they arrived, my fingers danced through the pages. I conjured kitchens from Tuscany to China and from stainless steel to granite. Colors swirled in my head, and I went to bed dreaming of paint and plaster.

The next day I started on the bathrooms. I imagined an opulent master bath in shades of royal purple and gold. Having chosen a Chinese theme, I threw in a few dragons and foo dogs.

Then, all excited, I sat my husband down and said, "Close your eyes and imagine this," and went into my delicious bathroom description.

When I said, "Can you see it?" his response was, "Ahh, nope. I only see black, and the inside of my eyelids."

Shocked, I realized that the man I married had no imagination! This set me on a path to discover what makes the imagination work. For me, it's pretty easy; I'm an artist and accused daily of having a wild imagination. I never thought about how I acquired my imagination or how it works until the day I discovered my husband didn't have one.

When you use your imagination, you tap into the divine part of your humanity. Imagination is the process of using all your senses to create a visual image in your brain, which has the ability to become matter in your life—it is how you create your reality. If you cannot imagine it, the "it" cannot exist. Having a healthy imagination is the doorway to a healthy mind, body, and spirit. If you can imagine good health, you can have it. Your imagination is just like a muscle; it can be developed and strengthened, and the more you use it, the wilder it will become. The foundation for any visualization or manifestation program is the ability to imagine. From that foundation you can create a life from which all good things flow.

"There is only one admirable form of the imagination:
the imagination that is so intense it creates a new reality,
that it makes things happen."
—Sean O'Faolain, 1900–1991

It amazes me how the primary part of creating a good life is stifled in so many of us at a young age. We are told that daydreaming is bad. We are scolded in school. What is even more amazing is that centuries ago poets, artists, and musicians had patrons who would cover their expenses just so they could daydream! They were encouraged to imagine. They spent the season in the country, in perfect creative communities. On a country estate, on a sunny day in May you could find George Sands, Fredric Chopin and friends sitting under a tree exercising their "imagination muscles"! From picnics and long candlelit dinners filled with wild conversations, the novels, concertos, poems, and paintings we enjoy today were created.

When was the last time you just had a conversation about your latest, greatest idea? When was the last time you had a great idea? My favorite ad is a picture of the seashore where someone has carved into the sand, "I am your idea. One day you'll look for me and I'll be gone." Is a wave about to crash onto the shore, washing away your idea?

"If you can imagine it, you can achieve it. If you dream it, you become it."

—William Arthur Ward, 1921–1994

So, how do you exercise this imagination muscle? How can you create your own reality? Start by playing with your senses.

Stress can inhibit imagination. So to relieve stress and set the stage to birth your imagination, find a soft spot, sit down, take three deep breaths, and play Mozart in the background. Think of the best memory you have, then write it down or talk to someone you trust. Use every descriptive word you can to recreate the memory, making up words for how it felt if there are no existing words to describe what you experienced. Is it Christmas or Chanukah? Is it your birthday, a day at the circus, or your first kiss? Describe the memory by using your senses. What did you hear? What did it smell like? What textures did you feel? What were the fragrances? What did you eat?

Imagination is activated and increased with the use of each additional sense. The stronger the memory the more your senses were affected during the occasion. Think about the month of December. The whole month creates a sensory experience. Touch is affected by ribbon and wrapping paper; sight is affected by the lights, garlands, and bright colors; sound is affected by laughter, song, and the music of the season; taste is affected by cookies, turkey, and all the trimmings; and scent is affected by the garlands, the tree, and the baking. Now choose your favorite memory and describe it using your senses.

"Memory feeds Imagination."

—Amy Tan, 1952–

Finished? How do you feel? Each day, when you are ready to work on your imagination, start with setting the stage to get your imagination cooking! My process of strengthening your imagination takes five weeks. It involves a little remembering, a little daydreaming, and a little playing with the senses. Each week we will be focusing on a different sense. The development of those senses will assist you in acquiring a wild imagination!

"Imagination grows by exercise and, contrary to common belief, is more powerful in the mature than the young."

—W. Somerset Maugham, 1874–1965

Week One—Focus: Sound

Supplies: *The Mozart Effect*™ CD (my favorite is *The Mozart Effect*™ Volume VI), CD player, and small tape recorder

Ever talk to yourself? Try it this week.

1. *Each day, remember to set the stage.* Find a soft spot, sit down, take three deep breaths, have the Mozart CD playing, and think about one of your favorite memories. Then use the "Ah" Meditation described below.

2.*The "Ah" Meditation.* Chant the sound "Ah" over and over. Try to stay focused on the sound for ten minutes. Listen to the sound of your breath and voice; listen to the way the sound moves through the room and vibrates through your body. When I first started doing this I chanted very softly, but by the end of the ten minutes I was yelling at the top of my lungs!

In Chinese medicine, sound is associated with the element of water, so listen to the sound of water in your life this whole week. Water also carries the energy of wisdom—accumulated philosophic, or scientific learning. During the next five weeks we will be gaining knowledge, having experiences, and growing in wisdom!

3. *Days one through four.* Have a little conversation with your imagination. Call on your imagination—your creativity—this week; ask it to show up! Tell yourself upon rising that you are highly creative and have a wild imagination. Say throughout the week, "Wow! I can imagine that!"

4. *Now think about your life.* How would you like it to change? Identify the desires, wants, longings, and hopes you are having trouble imagining, and we will work on them over the next few weeks. For simplicity, let's refer to them as "your dream." My definition of a dream is something that is real—a possibility within my reach that means I'm really cooking! Think about your dream as a real thing with no restrictions—emotional, spiritual, physical, or financial. You can have anything! Think about the dream in its completed, manifested form, not from the place of "Where do I start?"

My mom taught me how to do this when I was in the third grade. I decided to enter the school science fair and my project was "The Ear." I won a ribbon because of the way my mom helped me with my imagination. Her instructions were, "Think what the project looks like completed and work backwards. If you can imagine what it will look like in the end, you will figure out how to get there."

Try dividing your dreams in life into easy categories. In my workshops I call them the "Imagination Pages." The categories for me are: health, creativity, service, prosperity, and spirituality. Come up with your own categories—as many as you can think of—or borrow mine. For me, health includes my personal health; but it also includes the health of my family, friends, garden, house, animals, and my neighborhood. It gets bigger and bigger from there. Creativity includes any project I am working on, or anything I need to put energy into. The categories expand to fit what I am working on at the moment. Daydream, brainstorm, and think about what your dream is for three days.

5. *Day five.* Now that you have your dream defined, describe it using all the adjectives you can, making up words if you cannot find real ones to assist you. Say your dream out loud and listen to what the idea *sounds* like. When you love the way it sounds, tape it and play it back whenever you need a boost. The most effective way to begin the creative process is to use the checklist below:

a. Have you used the best, most positive language possible to describe your dream?

b. Recognize that when you use words like desire, need, want, wish—these words are *not* positive. They mean your goal is not something you have. And remember, I said you could have *anything*.

> Negative language is:
I hope to
I look forward to
I wish
I could
I would
> Positive language is:
I will
I have
I am

279

My husband was forty-five when we married and had never been married before. He had a good case of cold feet and everyone knew it! He actually had a temperature for three weeks after the wedding. We went to all kinds of doctors trying to figure out the source of the fever. Finally, the last doctor we consulted asked, "Has something stressful happened in your life in the last three weeks? Because you're perfectly healthy!"

The first two years after we married every time someone asked me, "How's it going? How's married life? How's he doing?" I would say, "I am happily married to the most grace filled man on earth. Today my friends and students who meet him say I am married to the most grace filled man they have ever met—he just seems so happy."

So make sure you use the most positive language you can. Go back and re-state the sentence so it carries the most positive energy possible. Really listen to what you say. Tape yourself, play it back, and let your language tell you where you are stuck. For example: "I could promise to commit to you," or "I really would like to" are statements that lack commitment. Make sure your language is strong and positive.

- List the pro and cons of your dream and see what is standing in your way
- Remember, you can have anything
- Focus only on the positive

6. *Day six.* Today appreciate sound in your life. Listen to *The Mozart Effect*™ CD; it is the best way to turn on your imagination! Mozart is *the man!* According to *The Mozart Effect* author Don Campbell, "His music has the best auditory components for stimulating the brain, relaxing the body, and creating a sense of order. Music can regulate brain function, language and speech development, modify posture, and create an emotional atmosphere that facilitates integration in the midbrain."

Don't know about the midbrain? Well, according to Dr. Joe Dispenza, author of *Evolving Your Brain: the Science of Creating Personal Reality*, "The midbrain is the first door to the subconscious. It assists us with the bonding process, whether that be human bonding like child and parent, or even bonding with concepts. It is the part of the brain that can also think in future time. Also known as the limbic brain,this primitive area about the size of an apricot sits right under the big thinking neocortex, and provides us with several mechanisms for survival as well. It is the home of the autonomic nervous system, which is the automatic nervous system. It regulates all those bodily functions that we don't have to consciously think about doing like controlling digestion, blood sugar levels, body temperature, and even emotions or feelings.

"Proper sounds in music can stimulate this part of the brain to make specific chemicals that make us feel good and blissful. The midbrain can also make chemicals that can make us feel angry, stressed or depressed. When this part of the brain is turned on, it makes the related chemicals equal to how we interpret our surroundings. It can act to support us by making us feel a certain way equal to our own personal thinking. You can compare the midbrain to an automatic factory of chemicals that facilitates our sensual responses to the environment or our own internal thinking. Through the limbic brain, great music can therefore entrain us to change our very feelings by changing our internal chemistry."

7. *Day seven.* Find a trusted friend to talk with about the experiences of your week. Own your experiences. Explain to your friend that he or she is not to judge, just listen to, the possibility of your dream. Describe the week and your creativity using all the words—all the adjectives—you can think of. Once again, make up words if you cannot find real words to assist you. See if you can make him or her see, feel, and taste the deliciousness of your first week of being highly creative!

"Go confidently in the direction of your dreams. Live the life you imagine."

—Henry David Thoreau, 1817–1862

Week Two—Focus: Sight

Supplies: *The Mozart Effect*™ CD, CD player, digital camera, magazines, photos, scissors, glue, crayons, plain white paper, and a blank photo album with paper pages for your "Imagination Album"

Did you ever see something you really wanted? Did you ever see your dream while driving around? This week, look for your dream everywhere you go, even on common errands. Notice everything. Become a detective for the life you imagine. Be prepared to capture your dream with your camera, so always have it by your side.

1. *Each day, remember to set the stage.* Find a soft spot, sit down, take three deep breaths, have the Mozart CD playing in the background, think about your favorite memory, and begin your "Ah" Meditation.

In Chinese medicine, sight is associated with the element of wood, so this week find your favorite tree. Wood also carries the energy of kindness—a state of being sympathetic or helpful in nature, to give pleasure or relief. Express yourself in kind ways this week to have a better understanding of the sense of sight.

2. *Days one and two.* Collect all your favorite magazines and photos and spend a few minutes each day cutting out pictures that relate to one of your dream categories. Make divisions in your album for each of your categories: health, creativity, etc., then cut and paste your pictures into your Imagination Album. When was the last time you got glue all over your fingers or played with scissors and crayons? Think you can't draw or color? Well, just take the crayon and scribble with wild abandon on the background of your pages, or scribble circles around your favorite picture on each page. Be six years old and have fun! (And I must encourage you to appreciate the wonderful fragrance of crayons here, even though I'm getting ahead of myself in the sense parade).

3. *Days three through seven.* Take your crayons and spill them out on the table. Close your eyes, mix them up, and roll them around. Open your eyes and quickly pick four crayons. Line them up in order of choosing. Each of the four colors will become a color of the day. On the morning of day four take your first choice and scribble on plain paper, going from one corner to the other, lightest to darkest. Try to get a wide range of the same color on the paper. This is the color of the day. Become the color, immerse yourself in the color, eat the foods of that color, and wear the color. Take a walk or drive (let someone else drive so you can just look out the window) and see how many shades of the color you can find. Do the same color exercise for days five, six and seven.

The first time I ever did this my family was on a long road trip and I had reached a level of boredom that had me staring out the window. All of a sudden green was everywhere! I lost count at twenty shades of green across the countryside. So during the rest of the trip, I divided the world by colors and kept track of how many different shades of each one showed up! Each day became a new color.

4. *Days one through seven.* Play the The Mozart Effect CD any time you want to get into a creative frame of mind.

5. *Any day during this week.* Go to the museum with a friend. Show each other favorite sights. If it is day 4-7, don't forget your color of the day. Describe your favorite sights using all the words— all the adjectives—you can think of and once again, make up words up if you cannot find real words to assist you.

6. *Days one through seven.* Practice "Candle Focus." Each night before bedtime, light a candle and focus on the candle's flicker light for five minutes. Stare at the flame and stay focused. Each time a distraction comes up, pull your focus back to the flame. Don't forget to blow out the candle before you go to sleep!

On day six, light the candle, focus on it, close your eyes, and imagine the flame—see it in your mind's eye. Open your eyes, focus on the flame, then close your eyes and imagine the flame. Do this five times in a row.

On day seven, go to the candle but do not light it—close your eyes and imagine that the candle is lit. See how long you can hold your focus!

One of my favorite stories about dreaming and the sense of sight is from Gene Sparling. Gene had been a bird watcher since he was young. He used to dream about finding a colony of ivory-billed woodpeckers. However, that variety of woodpecker had been extinct for sixty years; or so everyone thought until late winter 2004, when Gene spotted his dream bird while kayaking in the Cache River in Arkansas. No one believed him until a team of researchers from Cornell University met him on the river, and within 48 hours the ivory- billed woodpecker flew out in front of the team! He dreamed his woodpecker into reality. It took a while, but his dream came true!

Don't be afraid to go out on a limb .... It is where the fruit is!

—Anonymous.

Week Three—Focus: Taste

Supplies: *The Mozart Effect*™ CD, CD player, someone you trust to go to a Whole Foods Market or an Asian market, blinders, paper, and pencil.

In the evenings, continue the "Candle Focus" from week two.

1. *Each day, remember to set the stage.* Soft spot, sit down, take three deep breaths, play Mozart in the background, think about your favorite memory, and begin your day with the "Ah" meditation.

In Chinese medicine, taste is associated with the element of fire, so cook one of your meals on the barbeque or go to someplace where you can have grilled veggies. Fire also carries the energy of humility. Humility relates to being humble or reflective, so with each bite reflect with gratitude that there is a delicious meal on your table.

2. *Days one through seven.* This is a week of bravery. Be bold— eat a new fruit or vegetable each day this week. Go to the latest ethnic restaurant everyone is talking about.

My brother is a wonderful, brave, adventurous, single man who survives on white bread, mayonnaise, and bologna. He once had a dear friend visit from Mexico City. His friend wanted to take him out for an authentic Mexican meal, so off they went to the Hispanic section of Los Angeles. To enter into the spirit of the adventure, my brother allowed his friend to order. The unusual meal arrived shortly with nothing that my brother recognized or knew quite what to do with on his plate. His only experience with Mexican food to date was Tex-Mex with me in Dallas, and fajitas don't count as authentic. So looking at his plate and surrounded by the owner, all the waitresses, and his beaming friend, he began to eat a meal of very unfamiliar items, accompanied by what he described as "rice water" to drink.

Driving back to his office after lunch, he phoned his secretary, who is Hispanic, to ask what he had eaten. He described his meal saying, "Well, it looked like tongue and cactus, tasted like tongue and cactus, and went down like tongue and cactus." She confirmed his suspicion and said, "Yes, it was tongue and cactus!" By the time he returned to his office, she had somehow found a life-sized poster of a cow with its tongue hanging out of its mouth, and pinned it to his door!

When my brother found out about my imagination workshop, he said I should tell my students that if he could eat tongue and cactus, you folks should be brave enough to try a few odd fruits!

A TASTE ADVENTURE

Send your friend to Whole Foods Market or the Asian market and ask them to choose among the unusual fruits and vegetables that can be eaten raw. Have him or her choose things with texture that need to be peeled, and that have exotic fragrances. (Be responsible—let your friend know of any allergies you may have!)

Set aside some time when the two of you can spend about thirty minutes together and play with your sense of taste!

Set the stage and have pencil and paper available. Have your friend prepare a plate of the goodies out of your view, washed and ready for you to begin a tasting. Make sure you have not seen any of the purchases. Relax and put on your blinders and begin the process of feeling, smelling, and tasting your way through each item. Describe them, using all the words—all the adjectives—you can think of and once again, make up words if you cannot find real words to assist you.

My husband came to one of my workshops and he was great. While he was blindfolded, I handed him a tiny, Darling Clementine tangerine. When he described it, all the normal words came out first—tangy, tender, juicy, etc., and then out came "cartilaginous"! I was thrilled that he came up such an original word. I held the microphone to his mouth and asked for a definition and spelling. Still blindfolded and with a big smile on his face, he defined "cartilaginous" as the white, stringy, cartilage-like stuff surrounding the tangerine that needs to be removed before eating (by the way, it is a real word).

Being brave creates new neural connections in your brain. This stimulates and increases your imagination, providing you with new adventures and great stories to tell. Now to finish your week, go tell someone about your taste adventures!

"So you see, imagination needs moodling—long inefficient, happy idling, dawdling and puttering."

—Brenda Ueland, 1860–1985

Week Four—Focus: Touch

Supplies: *The Mozart Effect*™ CD, CD player, blinders, garden tools, fresh potting soil, flowers, lotion, someone you can massage, a bunny, a cat, a dog, and a human.

Continue the "Candle Focus" in the evenings.

Touch seems to be the most neglected sense, or the sense least appreciated. We are constantly touching clothes, the keyboard, the carpet under our feet, etc. We have become so accustomed to those things that we have stopped noticing the sensations they create. So, to be activated, touch has to be heightened. We seem to only notice touch if something uncomfortable happens, such as getting an ice cube down our shirt or burning our finger while cooking.

When I was in college I had the coolest art instructor; his name was Mr. Boggs. I was a very neat and tidy art student, but Mr. Boggs believed that a person had to loosen up and not be afraid to get dirty to be a really good artist. This man changed my life with his frustration about my being neat. Pottery was a required course, and when you are working on a potter's wheel it is impossible to stay clean. I would work a little while and wash my hands—I just did not like the way the clay felt drying on my hands. Mr. Boggs finally got frustrated with me and took both my hands, stuck them in a big trash can of clay, and made me play with it the whole period. By the end of the semester pottery was my favorite course. Today my primary art medium is clay!

1. *Each day, remember to set the stage.* Soft spot, sit, deep breaths, play the Mozart CD, think about your favorite memory, and begin your day with the "Ah" meditation.

In Chinese medicine, touch is associated with the element of earth, so this week have an earthy experience. Earth carries the energy of trust, which is assured reliance on the character or ability—the strength of someone or something. So this week, tell someone in your life that you trust what you have been up to with all this new wisdom you have gained. Experience trust—savor the experience of being in a secure place.

2. *Day one.* Today is for planting the yard, filling hanging baskets or pots with flowers for your porch, or re-planting something.

Set out all the tools, the potting soil, the flowers, etc. Close your eyes and feel each object—the cold and smoothness of the steel tools, the crumbly, warm earth, the tender, soft, velvet petals of the flowers. I always think it is important to own the experience, so tell someone about the pleasure of your planting day.

My greatest moments of divine connection have been when working in the garden—covered with mud, a little hot and sweaty, surrounded by the glory of nature; even if just moving plants to different pots, I love touching the soil and the plants, and feeling the sunshine on my face.

3. *Any day during this week.* This week, find time to give a massage to a loved one—a pet or human. I got a bunny for my last birthday—a glorious miniature bunny. He loves ear massages, and his nightly ear massage makes him do a "bunny purr." No matter how often my husband and I cuddle with him, the first thing we say is, "He's so soft." The texture of his fur reminds us on a daily basis of the beauty of touch. Most animals love an ear massage. Start at the base of the ear and work your way out to the ends, moving in small circles. Try a hand massage on your human loved one; get a little squirt of lotion and do the massage the same way. Start at the base of the fingers and slowly, gently work your way out to the ends of the fingertips.

4. *Days one through seven.* Make time for you! Get a dry brush massage. Call around and see who can provide you with this amazing feeling. A soft dry brush is rubbed all over your body. It has several purposes, including exfoliating the skin and stimulating the lymphatic system. But for our purpose, it is for you to feel the brush on your skin. It is one of the most interesting and pleasant massages you can imagine!

5. *Any day this week.* During one meal eat with your fingers—no napkins or utensils, just fingers! As with "finger-lickin' " chicken, just lick your fingers clean. Make sure you have dessert—something chocolate and gooey. Enjoy the texture of the food and feel the warmth. Loosen up, be a kid, dig in and enjoy yourself!

"Creativity represents a miraculous coming together of the uninhibited energy of the child with its apparent opposite and enemy, the sense of order imposed on the disciplined adult intelligence"

—Norman Podhoretz, 1930–

Week Five—Focus: Smell

Supplies: *The Mozart Effect*™ CD, CD player, one bottle of your favorite pure essential aromatherapy oil (try Whole Foods Market or a holistic/organic food store), another bottle of lavender pure essential oil, sixteen ounces of two percent fat milk, a new small paring knife, a lime, an orange, a grapefruit, a lemon, a tangerine or kumquat, a blender, citrus dishwashing liquid, a bucket, and a sponge.

Continue the "Candle Focus" in the evenings.

The easiest of the five senses to play with is smell. I find it interesting that smell is the strongest sense related to memory, and also the only sense described using different words. For example, "Do I smell something?" usually means something stinky. "What is that scent?" usually means something good. "Ah, the fragrance—" usually means something *really* good. These days scented items such as scented candles, air freshener, lotions, bubble bath, etc. have become a trend. Aromatherapy can be found everywhere, from grocery stores to gas stations. This week, instead of artificial scents, we are going to dive into the real thing. We are going to have a wide range of smelling experiences. Remember, smell can deceive—some of the worst smelling things can bring on the greatest delights!

1. *Each day, remember to set the stage.* Soft spot, sit, deep breaths, play the Mozart CD, think about your favorite memory, and begin your day with the "Ah" meditation.

In Chinese medicine, scent is associated with the element of metal, so buy a new paring knife for the experiment of the week. Metal carries the energy of integrity, which is firm adherence to a code, especially moral or artistic in value. This week look back over the last four weeks; come up with your own code of integrity to continue to develop your imagination.

2. *Days one and five.* Take a bath—not a regular one, a special one—an aromatherapy bath. Take one cup of two percent milk, put ten drops of your favorite pure essential oil into the milk, and pour it into your running bath water. Adding the oil to the milk

will give it the ability to disperse evenly throughout the bath, and is the easiest way to play with the oil.

3. *Any night this week.* When you can devote a night to good sleep, place four drops of lavender on a hanky, tissue, or wash-cloth. Slide it into your pillowcase and have a good snooze.

4. *House Cleaning Day.* Devote one day to cleaning your house, but make your own cleaning solution. Here is my homemade rec-ipe:

- Take the citrus fruits—lime, orange, grapefruit, lemon, tangerine or kumquat—and peel them
- Set the fruit aside
- Gather up all the peels, put them in a blender, add a little water, then puree
- Pour the puree into a bucket
- Add two quarts of water and a couple of squirts of dishwashing liquid
- Mix thoroughly

This is the most amazing way to clean the house. Use the solu-tion to wash the floor and counters. Ring out the sponge, shake off the peels, and clean away! It will be the most enjoyable cleaning experience ever. Play the Mozart CD really loud while you clean!

One day during the time my new husband was home with his fever and I was out at work, he came upon my cleaning mixture. I had prepared it early that morning for a friend who loved it, and then stashed it away in the 'fridge. Rooting around for something to eat, my sweet, fevered husband thought he had come across one of my famous soups, and decided to heat it up. I came in as the "soup" was bubbling, just in time to save him. So if you have any of the mixture left over, make sure you put a note on the con-tainer!

5. *Last but not least.* Okay, one last memorable experience! Go to the Asian market and buy a durian. In purchasing a durian, look for a yellow to brown skin, the heavier the better—a skin that is just beginning to split lengthwise! Fresh is always better than frozen. The durian is an unbelievable fruit with a rich, al-mond flavored, butter-like custard inside, and a prickly skin outside. It's shaped like a football and has an odd, amazing odor. The smell coming from this giant fruit is a combination of cream

cheese, onion sauce, and sherry. The more you eat it, the more you want it.

The durian has been said to be worth a voyage to the Far East to experience! One of the largest fruits in the world, it can grow to over ten pounds. It has high levels of tryptophan—the amino acid that helps alleviate depression by raising seratonin levels—tons of vitamin E, and one of the highest amounts of protein found in a fruit! It is one thing that fills every requirement of an imaginative experience—the skin is prickly to the touch, the taste is like the best pudding ever, the smell will knock you over, it is the strangest thing you have ever seen, and when you cut it open you will definitely hear a sound! It is an experience to be shared, so invite at least three friends over to assist you!

Your imagination is your greatest divine gift. It is the way God shows up in you. I challenge you to meet God and to experience the glory you can create. Be open to new adventures, new conversations, new tastes, new sounds, and new textures. If you will get out of your box—get out of your old habits and routines and expand—you will have a wild imagination!

I'll end the same way I started:

Imagine...

Imagine that you could manifest whatever you want.

"Whatever your mind can conceive and believe it can achieve."
—Napolean Hill, 1883 –1970

Imagine that that you could focus during meditations or visualizations.

"First comes thought: then organization of that thought into ideas and plans; then the transformation of those plans into reality. The beginning, as you will observe, is your imagination."
—Napolean Hill, 1883 –1970

Imagine that you could tap into your best and highest destiny.

"Everything you can imagine is real."
—Pablo Picasso, 1881 –1973

About The Author

Donna Collins

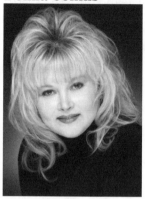

Donna Collins has dedicated herself to helping people live more creative lives utilizing her incredible imagination, creativity, and extensive knowledge of the Chinese art and science of feng shui. As an internationally recognized artist holding degrees in Art, Art History and Religion, Collins has combined her extensive art background with exhaustive studies of feng shui to produce a wide range of applications for her special talents. She is one of only six people in the world conferred the title of Master from the Mastery Academy of Chinese Metaphysics, the world's most prestigious feng shui educational institution. Her reach extends across the globe, including such clients as the Saudi Royal Family, Merrill Lynch, Southwest Airlines, and Toni and Guy, just to name a few. She has also enhanced her knowledge and resources through studies with the Dalai Lama, The HeartMath Institute, and the Ramtha School of Enlightenment. Collins has served on the board of various charitable organizations and was Executive Coordinator of the 2004 Gather the Women International Congress, which hosted forty non-profit organizations and United Nations partners from over twenty countries. Collins continues to inspire individuals, groups, and corporations to tap into their own intuition and creativity in all aspects of their lives, via one-on-one sessions as well as group educational venues.

Donna Collins
Email: pureenergy@sbcglobal.net

Chapter 17

Women's Mental Health

Vidushi Babber, M.D.

The Female Brain

Anatomical differences between men and women have existed since the beginning of time. However, scientific research has discovered that variations in the brain itself are present between the male and female eventually leading us to believe that this is probably why men and women "think" differently. Emotional reactions and behavior play a huge role in the thought process of both genders.

When examined closely, the female brain possesses a more active paralimbic cortex. This area is responsible for emotional reactions and is considered a highly evolved area of the brain. Maternal instincts and the so called "woman's intuition" are thought to originate from this particular location. Having an emotional connection with the outside world and being in tune with the needs of others, most likely provides the basis for why women are seen as more "sensitive" in comparison to men.

Aside from the composition of the brain, the body is also influencing the mind. Recent research has begun to identify the action of reproductive hormones in neurobiology. Estrogen and progesterone levels vary throughout a woman's life cycle thereby suggesting that the brain may be responding to factors other than the environment. The most critical stages of hormonal shift occur during the menstrual cycle, pregnancy, postpartum, and menopause. The combination of biological differences, environmental stress, and hormonal influence may motivate us to better understand why women are twice as more likely than men to suffer from mood disorders.

Menstrual Cycle

Premenstrual syndrome, commonly known as "PMS" has become the dreaded monthly phenomenon for some women. Although it is associated with normal ovarian function, the etiology of the emotional and physical symptoms is still unclear. However, there is strong evidence of hormonal influence on the brain leading to mood and behavior changes. These symptoms typically present before menstruation and subside after menses. The symptomatology can be grouped as physical, emotional and behavioral.

- *Physical Symptoms* include weight gain, hot flashes, headaches, abdominal cramps, bloating, fatigue, and breast tenderness.
- *Behavioral Symptoms* can be seen as isolation, decreased concentration, lack of interest in activities, and/or binging.
- *Emotional Symptoms* which may be experienced are feelings of depression, anxiety, irritability, anger or hostility.

Women who experience a severity of these symptoms interfering with their social and occupational functioning may be diagnosed with premenstrual dysphoric disorder or PMDD. This disorder is classified under a psychiatric condition known as "Depressive Disorder Not Otherwise Specified." Regardless of the classification, both PMS and PMDD occur in response to a hormonal and biochemical imbalance. Nearly seventy-five percent of women who menstruate suffer from PMS and almost four percent are diagnosed with PMDD.

This leads to a woman becoming susceptible to mood and anxiety disorders during later stages in her reproductive cycle. Studies have concluded that PMS may be a heritable condition and highly associated with stress in life. Furthermore, severity of symptoms during the premenstrual phase may predict difficulties during future critical stages in life where again hormonal shifts may occur such as pregnancy, postpartum, and menopause. PMDD can be diagnosed by daily rating of symptoms for at least two menstrual cycles. Women are asked to rate the severity of symptoms and chart them daily. This assists in identifying when the symptoms improve or worsen during the cycle. Appropriate interview and laboratory testing are required by a physician to rule out any other conditions which may have similar presentation to premenstrual problems.

Lifestyle changes are recommended in prevention of PMS. These include eating and exercising regularly, and limiting caffeine, alcohol, and salt intake. Some studies have concluded daily supplemental vitamin B6 of calcium and magnesium (Mg) supplements also are beneficial. Severe cases of PMS or women with PMDD may need future treatments with medications such as over-the-counter pain relievers, oral contraceptives, hormone intervention, and antidepressants.

Pregnancy

Pregnancy marks the stage of many emotions in a woman's life. Happiness and excitement are responses a mother is expected to experience. Unfortunately, this may not always be the case. Pregnancy also may be perceived as a stressful life event leading to psychiatric disorders which unfortunately are overlooked and often dismissed. The stress may begin as early as preconception when a woman is unable to become pregnant. Furthermore, should her pregnancy be confirmed, the thought of a healthy pregnancy becomes the focus. If a woman experiences any complications they may contribute to her anxiety and possibly even precipitate depression. These symptoms are often missed and therefore definitely need to be recognized early on as they may further complicate the health of both the mother and fetus.

During pregnancy, hormonal shifts are occurring which affect the brain. The body is preparing for the growth of the fetus, future nourishment, and feeding. As a result, levels of estrogen are varying during the pregnancy. This in turn affects a mother's mood stability. If one has a history of depression in the past, this state of increased estrogen level may cause a dysfunction possibly triggering another episode of depression. However, mood changes can also be seen for the first time during pregnancy—a time where the body is put under enormous stress in the process of preparing for a birth. During this period, hormones such as prolactin and progesterone are rising. Progesterone is being secreted from the placenta, which may contribute to depressive symptoms.

Throughout the pregnancy, levels of prolactin are gradually increasing as well. The rise may be linked to irritability or anger. Oxytocin and cortisol may also contribute to mood disturbance. What drives these mood changes is the inability of the brain to self-regulate the sudden shifts in hormonal levels. If the brain is able to in a way "keep up" with the pregnancy, mood stability is achieved by the middle of the pregnancy. However, if chemical/hormonal dysfunction continues, it may increase a woman's risk of experiencing further emotional distress.

Attention is crucial in pregnancy. Women need to be screened and if possible re-screened throughout a pregnancy for any changes in her mood. If left ignored, it may create further deterioration in the well-being of the mother and child in the future. Depression and anxiety will impact a woman's basic need such as eating, sleeping, etc., leading to complications in her pregnancy. As observers, we focus only on the growing body of the woman while she is pregnant but we fail to recognize the effect of the changing body on the brain and vice versa. We almost "forget" about the psychological impact and emotional difficulties in adjusting to motherhood. Pregnancy may be a happy time but it is definitely a stressful one, no doubt. Studies have produced evidence that deteriorating emotional health leads to premature labor, low birth weight, and premature infant births because the fetus receives fewer nutrients and less oxygen when the mother's body is under "stress."

Nearly twenty percent of women experience some symptoms in pregnancy of which ten percent develop a major depressive disorder. The prevalence of mood disorders has been noted to be similar to other times in a woman's life. However, symptoms may not always be identified; as a result, these women are left untreated.

When diagnosing mental illness in the pregnant population, it has become evident that the third trimester is when symptoms are reported most often. These symptoms may not meet the full criteria needed to diagnose a psychiatric disorder. This can possibly be due to the fact that the duration or number of symptoms may not be sufficient to make a clear assessment. It has been suggested that a screening tool may be necessary which accounts for the nature of the pregnancy and the deterioration caused by stress rather than trying to clearly define through the symptoma- tology outlined in specific criteria. These methods may incorporate self-report rather than an objective/subjective as- sessment made by a physician. The basis behind this approach originates from the limited time and exposure an office setting, which centers around the labs and examinations required in pre- natal visits. Regardless of the approach, it is mandatory that we be cognizant of the emotional well-being of a woman during her pregnancy and prevent any possible impairment in her mental health which again affects the outcome of the pregnancy.

Diagnosing depression may also sometimes be difficult given the disturbances of sleep, appetite, and energy changes, which also are part of pregnancy. Many women whose past history of mood disorders have experienced recurrent depression after dis- continuing their medication upon learning they are pregnant. In order to treat symptoms, several treatments are recommended. Forms of therapy suggested may include supportive, interper- sonal, and cognitive therapy. In addition, selected antidepressants have been known to be safe during pregnancy although most psychiatric medications are still being studied at this time.

Treatment is also dependent on the time in pregnancy when symptoms appear. Initially, during the first few months, there is concern about medication causing harm to the fetus. If the medi- cation is needed during this time, then it is most likely beneficial to continue throughout the pregnancy. Similarly, if treatment is initiated at any time during the pregnancy, treatment should be continued until several months postpartum toward the end of pregnancy.

However, preventative measures need to be emphasized in women who are known to be at risk for developing mood disor- ders. It is therefore important to be aware of past history, symptoms, and previous treatments. Monitoring of the pregnancy is certainly necessary as an ongoing effort to prevent future epi- sodes or intervene with treatment. At times, the safest option may be to continue with medication in order to reduce the risk of maternal or fetal impairments. Again, a physician and the mother must together make the decision about appropriate medication, especially when research is limited regarding its safety during pregnancy.

Severe cases of mood disorders may also require hospitalization. Risk of depression in mothers, if left untreated, increases alcohol and drug use. Mood disorders also create interpersonal difficulties within the home and disturbs interaction between the pregnant mother and her children. As a result, women are unable to focus on healthy lifestyle choices. It is therefore imperative that recognition of mental illness occurs as early as possible in the pregnancy.

Postpartum

The next stage of the reproductive cycle which may trigger another disturbance in hormonal shift is after the birth of a baby. Depression after childbirth can range from mild to severe. Almost eighty percent of women are known to experience the "baby blues" within three to five days after delivery. These symptoms include sleep disturbance, mood liability, tearfulness, difficulty bonding with the infant, fluctuation of appetite, and hostility toward others. The symptoms have no particular trigger or stressor. They also have no relation to previous history of psychiatric conditions. Typically the symptoms resolve within ten days. Treatment usually centers on emotional support and reassurance. Further evaluation is mandatory in assessing whether a mother meets criteria for a Major Depressive Episode. Symptoms need to persist for a period of at least two weeks to be diagnosed with this disorder. This postpartum depression is commonly seen within the first month of delivery and peaks approximately three to six months later. Therefore, the highest risk is greatest in the postpartum stage than any time during a woman's pregnancy. Nearly ten to fifteen percent of new mothers experience postpartum depression (PPD). One-quarter of women have had a previous diagnosis of depression and more than one-half have had a previous episode of postpartum depression in earlier pregnancies.

Recognition of mental illness is important during pregnancy and postpartum. Some symptoms may arise as early as the first or second trimester of pregnancy. Clinical features may include low mood, poor concentration, feelings of inadequacy, and thoughts of harming the baby. Unfortunately, these symptoms are so severe that they may interfere with functioning during daily activities. Both biological and psychosocial factors contribute to the onset of PPD. Hormonal fluctuations of estrogen and progesterone and their sudden decline after childbirth may play a role. Another less common cause may be an under-active thyroid gland after delivery. Postpartum depression may also have a genetic predisposition given the occurrence is higher in those women with relatives suffering from depression. Previous history of PPD is the most important risk factor of a woman in determining her susceptibility to a future episode. Depression during or before pregnancy is also a strong indicator of possible risk of experiencing depressive illness after childbirth. Ongoing pregnancy complications, marital discord, or lack of a support system may also increase a woman's risk of developing PPD. Therefore, identifying women early in their pregnancy is vital so that precautions can be taken. Close monitoring is necessary during and after the pregnancy as well. It is crucial that all health care providers as well as friends and family members act upon any evidence of emotional deterioration exhibited by a pregnant woman. Failure to adequately treat these women can lead to dreadful consequence for both the mother and the child. Significant impairment can occur between mother and infant interaction. Research has shown that PPD can have increased negative effects on the baby that may last until childhood. These include developmental delays as well as behavior and learning problems. Furthermore, it increases their susceptibility to developing mood disorders.

Therefore, early screening becomes a major necessity in identifying deterioration in the well-being of both mother and child. Routine screening is critical during the prenatal, antenatal, and postnatal visits. However, due to limited time and focus on the physical health, emotional wellness is often overlooked. Depression rating scales focused particularly on symptomatology of pregnant women need to be further developed and incorporated within a normal routine visit for women during and after their pregnancy in order to accurately identify if they are at risk. These screening tools should address previous history, support systems, and current stressors in addition to physical and emotional symptoms. Screening should also be occurring at regular intervals to determine the severity and need for intervention.

Several treatment approaches have been identified to help lessen the severity and prevent further deterioration. Although there is limited research, medications have proven beneficial during the postpartum period. However, if there is a mild case, psychological interventions of therapy and support groups have assisted women in overcoming their fears and depression. For moderate to severe cases, antidepressants have been used. The selective seratonin reuptake inhibitors (SSRI's) have been fairly safe throughout pregnancy during the postpartum period. Healthcare providers may recommend that women remain on these medications if they do have a history of depression, primarily as a preventative measure.

Psychosocial support is also crucial as it provides women with reassurance and hope. A mother may also question her ability to care for the infant during this time. Help provided by family or friends to assist with the transition to motherhood, therefore, is important. Should a woman's condition become severe and she experiences any psychotic or suicidal thoughts, hospitalization is necessary to assure her safety. Although the risk is minimal if adequately screened and proper treatment is provided in advance, it is not uncommon today to hear reports of cases in the media concerning women who harm themselves or their children after childbirth. Therefore, education and awareness needs to become an integral part of our society to ensure that together we not only minimize these occurrences but we eliminate the risk completely.

Menopause

Menopause marks the final period in a woman's life where the last hormonal shift occurs specifically due to the ending of ovulation. Nearly one-third of women in the U.S. have been through menopause. During this time, women experience both physiological and psychological symptoms. The relationship of menopause may be associated with biochemical changes such as fall in estrogen levels leading to destabilization of the mood. Women at this stage complain of symptoms of hot flashes, poor sleep, increased irritability, and anxiety. Menopausal transition psychologically affects women both positively and negatively. If a woman sees this change as a loss of fertility and has a negative view, she may experience more physical symptoms in addition to emotional difficulties. On the other hand, a woman who views menopause as more of a freedom or relief, tends to adjust to symptoms and experiences less difficulty in psychological adjustment of her menopause status. As a result, it becomes necessary to consider all aspects of a woman's life which may lead to her changes in mood. This perimenopause transition lasts anywhere from few months to a few years.

Risk seems to increase for those with a previous history of depression, postpartum depression, or PMDD. Therefore, a careful history of current and past symptoms needs to be taken. Appropriate exam and blood tests help assess the function of reproductive organs. Also, life stresses may be influencing a woman's susceptibility to mood disorders.

It is also important to recognize deterioration in memory during this phase in life. Studies have concluded that fall of estrogen is linked to poor memory and other cognitive functions. Further, this drop in estrogen affects a woman's ability to learn and process new information. When examining differences in the human brain, there is a faster decline in areas of the brain related to higher cognitive functioning such as the hippocampus. Researchers have questioned whether a lack of estrogen may be the reason this phenomenon occurs in the female brain after menopause. Moreover, studies have been conducted which have discovered improvements in learning and memory in postmenopausal women receiving hormonal treatments with estrogen thereby strengthening the theory of deficiency in estrogen causing cognitive decline.

Treatment options to manage mood symptoms related to menopause include antidepressants, psychotherapy, and hormonal treatments. Recommendations vary dependent on whether a woman is in the transitory phase or in complete menopause. The severity of the symptoms may also determine which treatment is best. Mild cases can be treated with either hormone replacement or antidepressants. If a woman is past the perimenopausal phase and there is cessation of menses, she is more likely to benefit from antidepressants for her mood symptoms. However, hormone replacement does provide health benefits other than improving depression. Physical symptoms such as night sweats, hot flashes, and insomnia may be relieved by hormonal therapy. Severe cases of depression can be treated by both antidepressant medication and hormone replacement. This may include a combination of estrogen/progesterone or only estrogen. Psychotherapy is highly recommended for depressive symptoms. Both cognitive behavioral and interpersonal therapy have been also suggested as treatment options for menopausal women diagnosed with depression.

Conclusion

As we have learned more about each stage of a woman's repro-ductive cycle, we better understand how these changes affect the emotional and mental state. We need to look past the stigma of mental illness as being a weakness of character and appreciate the hormonal and biological influences. After all, psychiatric ill-ness is a medical condition. Once we have embraced the importance of emotional well-being as much as a healthy body, we can as a society lend the support and understanding to those in need of care. As family members and friends, we need to accept that mental illness exists and through love and patience, we can enrich our lives with healthy minds...whether it be a man's or woman's.

About The Author

Vidushi Babber, M.D.

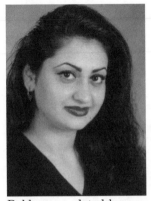

Vidushi Babber, M.D. currently serves as a Medical Director for the Adult Psychiatry Unit at Lake Charles Memorial Hospital. She is also in private practice at the Institute for Neuropsychiatry in Southwest Louisiana. Her expertise is in women's mental health issues for adolescents, adults, and the elderly. Dr. Babber received her Bachelor of Science degrees in Biology and Psychology from Houston Baptist University. She earned her Medical Degree at St. George's University School of Medicine. Dr. Babber completed her psychiatric training at Loyola University Medical Center in Illinois and University of Texas Medical Branch in Galveston, Texas. Dr. Babber also completed a Fellowship in Women's Mental Health at the University of Illinois in Chicago. Dr. Babber has received media training from the Texas Society of Psychiatric Physicians. In addition, she has completed a certified training course with the Professional Woman Network and is a part of their speaker's bureau. Dr. Babber has been awarded teaching honors for her work with students. She has been selected to present for several conferences, quoted in newspapers and interviewed on television. Her recent publication includes a book review on *The Postpartum Effect: Deadly Depression in Mothers.* She is an active volunteer in educating the community advocating the improvement of women's mental health through prevention and education. Dr. Babber is available for presentations on a local, national, and international basis.

Vidushi Babber, M.D.
Email: drbabber@yahoo.com

303

Chapter 18

Fat Chance At Last—
How to Go Beyond Willpower

Eileen Silva, Ph.D., N.D.

In the final analysis—after considering all the "best" lifestyle choices you could possibly make, weighed against the health issues you are dealing with—if you're like ninety-nine percent of the people I've worked with during the last thirty-five years, then you'll probably wind up thinking, "Fat chance!" That's why I've dedicated my career to the pursuit of health by going *beyond* willpower (which generally fails us when we most need it), and turning instead to the magic of body chemistry correction.

Operating like a forensic detective on a crime scene, and seeing the unseen, my role is to help you collect obscure clues and telltale signs of body chemistry imbalances, to offer you an easy blueprint for health you can follow for the rest of your life, while applying health tips already made available in this book by my esteemed colleagues.

The first thing for you to get clear about is that there *is* life after a health breakdown. Sometimes a health crisis can be a great wake-up call, even a life-changing defining moment. My own journey towards better personal health actually began more than thirty years ago, after receiving a diagnosis of an incurable illness, followed by about a decade of ineffective treatments and general health decline.

When I finally got on the road to recovery and eventually re-stored my health to better than it had been before my illness, my first inclination was to avoid health issues altogether and to focus on vitality and living. Then I realized I had a real passion to reach out to others who were experiencing the isolated feeling that no one could understand what they were going through and to help people reverse health issues as I did by balancing body chemistry, thus allowing the body to return to wellness. This process demystifies illness and empowers those who are really seeking a "healing field."

Actually, finding a "healing field" is a key to wellness. No mat-ter how brilliant the health professional may be, it is vital for the patient to trust and believe in the care and advice being given. When a healing field is created by this bond, then the body does have the capacity to heal from within, no matter how unlikely this might seem to the uninitiated.

Healing must always be created from within. That is not to say, of course, that products, medicines, foods, procedures, and the like are not to be considered. What it *does* mean is with the proper attitude, healing is an inside job. Part of the role of a healer is to be a good listener of both the said and the unsaid and to allow the patient to reveal important clues for consideration.

I remember doing a radio talk show for a station in Canada some years ago. It was one of those fun shows where listeners can call in live to ask the guest questions. I shared my own health crisis at the beginning of the show, and then we spent perhaps twenty or thirty minutes discussing little-known clues to immune health management. I soon had a caller who shared on the air that she had been to various doctors for almost a decade without a firm diagnosis, but was told she possibly had a lupus problem. Interestingly, as a former lupus sufferer, I know that if you have a possible lupus diagnosis, then you have a probable "lupus-like syndrome," which is actually a major immune dysregulation prob-lem masquerading as an autoimmune problem. According to environmental medical specialist, Dr. Jeffrey Anderson, nineteen out of twenty people who are diagnosed with lupus do not have a true case of the disease—they have a manifestation of it, coupled with general chronic illness symptoms. The normal and custom-ary treatment may actually be the wrong approach altogether. This is a frustrating situation for doctor and patient alike.

Right after I went off the air, the caller rang up my office number and asked for a long-distance consultation. Shortly after we completed that and got her going in a previously unexplored direction—treating this as a body chemistry imbalance instead of an illness—she experienced a major breakthrough.

"I feel like I've got totally different insides!" she exclaimed after only a week of a new protocol. She went on to have a complete remission from her previously chronic symptoms. For me, that is the reward for what I do. I know from my own previous frustration with traditional medical approaches that when you have a gloom and doom prognosis with no cure or effective treatment, and your day-to-day energy levels are poor, it is hard to be optimistic.

So, part of my commitment to my clients, and to you, is to open up the possibility that we all could enjoy a breakthrough healing. While there is life in your body it is never too late to make a huge difference with a new approach—a new or renewed faith—that all things are possible with God's help. No matter how bleak your prognosis has been, I totally believe that it is possible to send any disease into remission if you could effectively cleanse, balance, and oxygenate. The trick is—this is easier to say than to do. But aren't all good things worth working for, and aren't we all here to learn the lessons such a process can reveal to us?

My own decade-long convoluted journey back from my devastating health crisis eventually became the best thing that had ever happened to me. It taught me many lessons about seemingly unrelated things and revealed the importance of the mind in the recovery process. It also unveiled a purpose for my life that went far beyond anything I ever imagined, or even felt comfortable pursuing. For that reason, over the years I have expanded my intake process to include a 110-question multiple-choice questionnaire. This generates a customized twenty-two-to thirty-page color bar graph "snapshot" of the client's body chemistry in ten major areas, including stress imbalances, energy levels, colon toxicity, liver toxicity, yeast imbalance, mineral needs, dietary imbalances, metabolic slowdown, possible allergies, and body imbalances.

The computer-generated profile also provides a correct water formula and Body Mass Index (BMI), including probability charts for coming down with major degenerative health issues, based on medical statistics for those BMIs. It is then possible to get health baselines, which give us a very revealing starting point for creating improvements.

My interest has gone far beyond that of simply "fixing" health issues; I want to empower you to design an effective wellness blueprint for your life that involves a way of thinking as well as a way of being. The key is gaining insights to your real underlying health issues.

It's pretty amazing to me that my developing a computerized technology to make my consultations more consistently helpful—especially to those who wanted long distance support—has now evolved into my developing and conducting integrative wellness certification programs for medical doctors, as well as for chiropractors and doctors of naturopathy. That movement really picked up unsolicited steam when Dr. Harold Schulman, world-respected obstetrician/gynecologist, Einstein University medical instructor, author of more than 150 American Medical Association research papers and expert court witness, gave my program an unsolicited endorsement in one of his books as well as in his practice before he retired.

Through the influence of Dr. Schulman and others, I found myself smack-dab in a role I had never in my life imagined: catalyst for integrative medicine with a simple turnkey approach that the staff can run. This allows a caring doctor to once again become the manager of his patients' health care by having low-risk healthy options available to them as a logical starting point for those so inclined. With more than sixty-five percent of all medical dollars spent last year spent in *alternative* medicine (typically outside of the patient's primary care physician's awareness and insurance coverage), what was once considered controversial has now gone mainstream. You have probably sensed this in your own medical community, and you may have even had such a consultation locally—I hope so.

One of the health issues I have frequently encountered throughout the years with this process of total body analysis is a combination of high stress levels accompanied by low energy. Often this is coupled with insidious increasing weight gain. You can immediately assess your current metabolic performance by completing this quick, self-scoring health inventory.

The Twelve Trigger Questions for
MetaThermasis™ Inventory

1. Have you been on three or more diets in the last five years? _____NO _____YES

2. Have you gained more than five pounds in any six-month span of time since you were eighteen years old? _____NO _____YES

3. Do you tend to bloat after eating? _____NO _____YES

4. Are you sometimes or often water retentive? _____NO _____YES

5. Do you sometimes suffer from constipation or diarrhea? _____NO _____YES

6. Are you over twenty-five years of age? _____NO _____YES

7. Do you exercise fewer than three or more times per a week and/or find yourself under noticeable stress frequently? _____NO _____YES

8. Do you suffer from frequent fatigue and/or fail to "bounce" out of bed in the morning? _____NO _____YES

9. Do you eat fast foods once or more a week? _____NO _____YES

10. Do you drink less than eight full glasses of pure water per day? _____NO _____YES

11. Have you taken three or more over-the-counter or prescription drugs in the last three years? _____NO _____YES

12. Do you crave breads and/or sweets? _____NO _____YES

TOTAL NUMBER OF "YES" ANSWERS:

Scoring:

- Two or more "YES" answers indicates possible **MetaThermasis**™ slowdown
- Three to six "YES" answers indicates probable **MetaThermasis**™ slowdown
- Seven to twelve "YES" answers indicates definite **MetaThermasis**™ slowdown

PLEASE CHECK ALL THE CHALLENGES YOU WOULD LIKE TO OVERCOME:

- Cellulite
- Skin Tone
- Stress
- Bloating
- Junk Food Craving
- Exercise

- Appetite
- Water Retention
- Inch Gain
- Constipation
- Sugar Craving
- Weight Gain

- Uncontrolled Hunger
- Fatigue
- Loss of Muscle or Firmness
Other

My Three reasons for becoming healthier:

1. _____
   _____
   _____

2. _____
   _____
   _____

3. _____
   _____
   _____

Feel free to forward your **MetaThermasis** Survey results to Dr. Eileen Silva at the Hegan Center, 501 San Juan Drive, Suite "P," Southlake, TX 76092, or email it to ensilva@aol.com if you would like to review it with me.

By now, perhaps you are realizing your metabolism is not what it once was. Eventually, sluggish metabolism will result in weight increase accompanied by a general health decline. This is even more predictable for perimenopausal and menopausal women. There seems to be a round-robin effect; if women enter perimenopause in an overweight condition, they tend to be much more symptomatic, and they tend to gain even more weight. You see, gaining weight is not a problem—it is a *symptom*—a symptom of health imbalance.

If you have found your weight increasing throughout the years, one of your most significant unaddressed issues could be the presence of unknown parasites (including bacteria). While we need "good" bacteria in our system, most of us have an unhealthy proportion of undesirable bacteria called candida albicans (internal yeast). We end up with too much candida albicans primarily through the use and overuse of antibiotics as well as with the consumption of non-organic meat and dairy products heavily laced with antibiotics. Some of the common signs of a candida albicans imbalance include:

- vaginitis in women
- fatigue
- depression
- diarrhea
- thrush (oral or vaginal)
- constipation
- numbness
- persistent or recurring sore throat

- endometriosis
- bloating
- muscle tightness or weakness
- allergy
- memory lapses
- nasal congestion
- irritability
- swollen or painful joints

- athletes foot
- chemical sensitivities
- heartburn
- blurred vision
- headaches
- inability to focus and concentrate abdominal pain

In fact, possibly a more reliable clue of the presence of an unhealthy proportion of candida albicans is if symptoms are aggravated by damp weather, a moldy environment, or consuming sugar-rich foods or foods containing fungus. Situations that predispose one to a candida albicans imbalance include: pregnancy, a history of taking birth control pills, diabetes, having been on a cortisone or antibiotic regimen, having a history of prolonged illness, medication consumption, malnutrition, poor diet, an acidic pH, or a history of multiple types of allergies. In other words, if you have had health challenges, chances are pretty good that an internal flora imbalance is exacerbating your situation. An interesting note: a classic sign I look for is a person with a candida albicans imbalance who is a "reluctant" weight loser and easy weight gainer, the "I-gained-six-pounds-over-the-weekend" type.

I have found that, while theoretically, the commonly used "yeast connection" approach of strict dietary adherence to a candida starvation protocol, possibly combined with some candida-killing treatment, should work, it seldom provides any lasting results, and I will tell you why. I asked Dr. Russell Manuel, one of my *Fat Chance at Last!— How to go Beyond Willpower* book endorsers who taught immunology in six countries, "What happens when they quit following the strict regimen?"

"Oh, they can't do that," he said, "or it will come right back!"

"So, what have you really fixed?" I asked. He had no answer.

The regimen that I developed provides lasting change because it actually addresses the internal environment of the body more comprehensively by focusing on the body's pH and other issues that will be critical for success. Protein, for example, is the most acidic-producing food you could possibly eat; yet ironically, most traditional candida albicans eating regimens rely heavily on protein consumption.

Think of it this way: if your body were a room, and if we painted the room black, put in a strobe light, and brought in a few drug dealers, then we would attract a certain type of clientele to the room. If we re-decorated and painted the walls white, added stained glass windows, church pews, a pulpit and a pastor, then we'd attract a totally different clientele base. This is the concept of internal body atmosphere and the importance of understanding the ramifications of it if we want to alter body chemistry results.

My program consists of a brief, inexpensive but effective ten-day rejuvenation routine. It differs from the traditional approach in that it alters the pH toward alkalinity, strips excess mucous from the system, stimulates the energy flows in the body, cleanses very aggressively—including both the liver and the colon—addresses poor gut function issues, and it also involves a personal attitude of wellness expectation. Remember, thoughts *are* things, and it is important that our confidence in our ability to heal from within is strong.

Perhaps you have struggled with your flora balance for the very same reason as those who have followed the traditional approach for candida issues. You might have addressed some commonly supported challenges, while other factors that are important but more obscure have gone without being addressed. There may be up to 8,500 forms of parasites that could potentially live in the human body, based on temperature, pH, etc. The signs and symptoms of parasite infestation include fatigue, sugar cravings, bread cravings, poor complexion, hunger a short time after eating, or restless sleeping. Parasite issues can be a minor annoyance that simply impair our well-being in general ways, or parasite infestation can result in major body system malfunctions. Think about it: if you have unwanted parasites at work in the pancreas, wouldn't that issue be liable to interfere with pancreatic function?

Similarly, colon toxicity is very prevalent in America. When you combine the typical junk food Western diet with the stress levels people often experience, the average person is carrying around seven to twenty-five pounds of debris in the colon. Elvis Presley was said to have had sixty-two pounds of fecal matter in his colon upon autopsy. Colon toxicity is responsible for unwanted body odor, like bad breath. It can also be responsible for that protruding tummy that women tend to get below the waist. Common signs of colon toxicity include:

- overweight
- headaches
- irritability
- menstrual problems
- fatigue
- nervousness
- insomnia
- skin problems
- depression
- food cravings

- malaise
- protruding or even distended abdomen
- bad breath/body odor
- indifference
- leg swelling
- abdominal discomfort

- neuritis/neuralgia (chest pains)
- gas (upper or lower)
- anxiety/worry
- inability to concentrate
- loss of memory/mental confusion
- sex drive issues

Other possibilities, which doctors might note in people exhibiting autointoxification because of colon toxicity, are:

- coated tongue
- pot belly
- anemia
- malnutrition
- low blood pressure
- dark circles under eyes

- sallow complexion
- low blood pressure
- fetid breath

- high blood pressure
- cold hands/feet brittle nails & hair

In the early 1990s, while conducting a body balancing seminar in Atlanta, Georgia, I talked extensively about colon toxicity issues. After I finished my talk, a woman came right up to me and asked me if I had ever heard of colonics. "Oh yes," I assured her, "I've had them myself."

She went on to share an astonishing story with me about her own recent colonic experience. "I'm fifty-four years of age," she said, "and while I've eaten a lot of fiber and done a number of colon cleansing regimens, I recently I had a colonic for the first time. When the colon therapist was done with the procedure, he asked me when I had a barium treatment. I told him that I only had one barium treatment—when I was four years old. I then asked him how in the world he knew about it. He told me that he could always detect it because it deposits a gray clay-like coating to the colon that is not removed from normal fiber consumption." She went on to tell me that her daughter, who was in her thirties, had a barium treatment once when she was seven years of age. Since she was skeptical about the barium story, she told her daughter to go have a colonic, but not to mention anything ahead of time to tip the guy off. She finished her colonic, and the therapist said nothing. She decided to have another one, and at the end of the second colonic, the therapist asked, "When did you have barium?"

It makes sense, based on the commonness of the aforementioned colon toxicity clues, for you to do some work on colon cleansing as a preventive measure. Years before it became fashionable, Dr. Alvenia Fulton used to say, "Life and death begin in the colon."

One very logical way to approach cleansing is by making sure that you take in the proper amount of water each day. I define water this way: if you wouldn't wash your hair with it, you can't wash your cells with it. Water, therefore, is not orange juice, minestrone soup, or iced tea—water is water. Your optimal water formula is two quarts of water for all adults, plus an extra eight ounces for every twenty-five pounds or fraction of twenty-five pounds that you need to lose. So for most adult Americans, the correct water formula is about two and a half quarts of water per day. You also need more water if your health is less than optimal. A classic sign of dehydration is leg cramps.

One of the most thought-provoking incidents of my career occurred about ten years ago in Detroit. I was presenting a seminar on body balancing to a rather large audience—nearly 500 attendees. A very overweight woman came up to me at the conclusion of the program and asked for a private audience. I will call her "Lynn" for the purpose of anonymity. At first glance I could see Lynn seemed mentally disoriented, so I asked her husband to join us for note-taking. She told me she had driven six hours from Ohio to hear me speak, and that I was her last hope. She had experienced diarrhea for four straight years and *nothing* had worked for it, including an evaluation by the Mayo Clinic. Lynn also shared a heart-wrenching story of all the weight control programs she had tried and the underlying theme of those efforts. It seems she would begin a program with some initial weight drop but, shortly after its inception, she would begin to ooze a foul-smelling oily substance from her pores, especially in the hip area.

Not only was this a hideous embarrassment to her, but it was also disconcerting to the various doctors assigned to the clients. Without exception, each one had asked her to accept a refund and discontinue their program. Strange as it may seem, no one wanted to acknowledge any connection between their protocols and her disorder. Several doctors did send her on for more tests, but nothing ever showed up. I found that hard to believe, so I pursued asking Lynn about the testing. "You mean *nothing* abnormal ever showed up?" I demanded to know.

"Well no, not really," she said. She went on to explain that there was so much fecal matter obstructing the x-rays that they revealed nothing. I suggested a very tame protocol for her to begin—if her doctors had no objections—starting with drinking a gallon of pure water a day with fresh lemon juice in it for the first three days. Lynn looked at me like I was nuts and repeated to me that she had constant diarrhea and could not possibly drink a gallon of water a day on top of her other fluids. I made sure her husband was writing down the conversation, and then told her that since she had suffered with diarrhea for four years already, had gone to the Mayo Clinic, etc., it was reasonable for her to give me four weeks to evaluate the results of another "first do no harm" direction. "After all, the diarrhea is ongoing, so what do we really have to lose?" I asked her. Additionally, I pointed out to her that colon toxicity specialists consider diarrhea and constipation to be flip sides of the same problem.

Dr. Bernard Jensen, D.C., in his book, *Tissue Cleansing Through Bowel Movement*, says that over seventy million Americans are suffering from bowel problems. He throws in a thought-provoking quote from the American Cancer Society, "Evidence in recent years suggests that most bowel cancer is caused by environmental agents. Some scientists believe that a diet high in beef and/or low in fiber is the cause."

Not wanting to alarm Lynn, but needing to impress the gravity of the situation, I also mentioned that Dr. John Kellogg noted that many operations have been prevented by cleansing and revitalizing the bowel, and in his opinion, perhaps as much as ninety percent of all disease is due to improper colon function.

Lynn was skeptical, but desperate, so therefore willing. I was, she repeated, her last hope. We didn't have to wait long. After four long painful years of diarrhea, her problem cleared in four short days with the water regimen. When she called a week later to share the phenomenon and to thank me, she cried so hard that she could hardly speak. Thankful, but bitter about all the wild goose chases, she had this to say, "I can't believe that for four years I had constant diarrhea, that I've been to dozens of doctors and endured many tests, including a round at the Mayo Clinic, that I've taken everything every doctor ever prescribed to try to fix this and the answer was something as basic and free as *water*. No one at any time during the more than $10,000 worth of visits I've had has ever asked me about my water drinking habits. I am *so* angry!"

My counsel was to focus on the miracle we were experiencing. After all, my work is based in the logic of the "Big Picture" as I call it, and sometimes specialists are so involved looking at isolated body parts that the presentation of the entire body never enters in. I also pointed out that with $10,000 worth of tests and visits, she probably would not have welcomed a prescription from one of the medical experts to go home and drink water. As a footnote to her study, Lynn kept in touch with me for several years and did not relapse, except briefly, when travel prevented her from doing her water formula. She found that when she traveled, simply returning to her regimen almost immediately resulted in a dissipation of symptoms.

If your system is functioning at peak performance, then you aren't concerned at this point because you are having a bowel movement after every meal. But, what do you do if you are in that vast group of people whose systems don't function at that level?

You will want to visit my websites (www.eileensilva.com, www.dreileensilva.com, www.rxhealthlink.com) to download special health reports and information related to this issue. Here are some other guidelines for your immediate consideration:

1.   Be sure you are drinking your water formula (given earlier).
2.   Be sure your diet contains enough fiber, enzymes, and recommended daily allowances of nutrients.
3.   Avoid known allergens, especially food sources.

4.   Go on an aggressive cleansing regimen. Realize that if you were a car, we could drive you out into the driveway and clean you thoroughly in a few minutes, but you have miles and miles of convoluted pipes, so the process will take months, or possibly years, to correct lifelong build-up.

5.   Colon toxicity is the source of breath and body odor problems for most people. In fact, for all the millions of dollars Americans spent last year on mouthwashes, most represented just a short-term cover-up of a problem that was emanating from the colon. Those who wake up with "morning breath," touted by advertisers as the worst breath of the day, need to begin correcting the problem from the bottom up, so to speak.

6.   Try to reduce tension.

7.   Don't delay the urge when it strikes.

8.   Use digestive enzymes to help you break down foods better and to improve transit time.

9.   Consider having "pressure point" therapy or reflexology done on your hands, feet, and or ears to help the body heal and cleanse itself.

In the final analysis, how effectively you can stave off the aging process and maintain optimal health is largely up to you. When you are younger than fifty, good genetics and a little luck can help you look younger and feel better than you deserve, in spite of lifestyle abuse. We all know those people—the guy you went to high school with who smokes, eats fast food every day, drinks too much, fails to exercise, and is sleep deprived, but he looked good, until he hit the magic age of fifty, give or take a few years. For virtually all of us, after that defining moment, we begin to get the body and face we deserve. If we have neglected to exercise, we will definitely lose our muscle tone and flexibility.

As we began this book with some of Dr. Deepak Chopra's classic wisdom, perhaps it would be appropriate to repeat the importance of serving others so that we are able to maintain the sense of peace and well-being that only comes from making a contribution to those whose lives we touch.

When my health was threatened over three decades ago, I found that going back to examine roadblocks to my energy helped me see that lack thinking and negativity were a poor starting point for recovery. This is why, when I designed my computerized health analysis, I included those ten major body system issues with color bar graphs and hundreds of customized lifestyle management suggestions for the client. It's not just about what you take or do. It is really about who you are as a person and the healing energy you can create for yourself through making the mind/body connection, selecting better lifestyle choices, and correcting body chemistry issues. My belief is that you don't need to understand all of those body chemistry imbalances and you don't need to overanalyze them—you don't need to spend years in pursuit of their complexities.

What you *do* need to do is to become pro-active about your health. When you partner with your health practitioners and take responsibility for how you feel, then you are on the right track. If you want further customized insights about your health, my consultation is a one-time experience that takes place over the telephone. It is a very affordable opportunity for you to assess where you are and what your healthy options include. You may not need that at all—you might instead just decide if you are ready to invest some energy into applying the phenomenal insights my colleagues have provided in this book.

Think about it: if you knew that the next French fry you ate was going to kill you, would you eat it? And yet, many of us have continued with lots of those bad habits expecting different results. Isn't it time to take charge and to stop deluding yourself? Isn't it time to *really* go beyond willpower... and to unlock the secrets to creating a healthier you?

Eileen Silva, Ph.D., N.D.

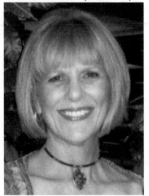

Eileen Silva, Ph.D., N.D., is a doctor in Natural Health and Naturopathy, in Southlake, Texas, with a practice in metabolic health, weight, and body balancing. As CEO of Hegan Center, Eileen has trained and certified medical doctors and chiropractors for almost a decade. Her innovative wellness techniques have been used to help thousands of individuals achieve weight loss and better fitness. Additionally, Eileen's programs have brought enhanced energy, weight balance, and longevity to professionals in corporate wellness programs. Eileen is an active member of the American Naturopathic Medical Association, the American Holistic Health Association, the Health Sciences Institute, and the National Speakers Association. She has been treating patients and teaching workshops on integrative medicine for over 18 years.

Dr. Eileen Silva
Phone: 817.424.5204
Email: Eileen@DrEileenSilva.com
www.dreileensilva.com
www.rxhealthlink.com
www.eileensilva.com